NONLINEAR PEDAGOGY AND THE ATHLETICS SKILLS MODEL

This book offers an ecological conceptualisation of physical literacy. Re-embracing our ancestry as hunter gatherers we gain a new appreciation and understanding of the importance of play, not only in terms of how children learn, but also in showing us as educators how we can lay the foundations for lifelong physical activity. The concept of physical literacy has been recognised and understood throughout history by different communities across the globe. Today, as governments grapple with the multiple challenges of urban life in the 21st century, we can learn from our forebears how to put play at the centre of children's learning in order to build a more enduring physically active society.

This book examines contemporary pedagogical approaches, such as constraints-led teaching, nonlinear pedagogy and the athletic skills model, which are underpinned by the theoretical framework of Ecological Dynamics. It is suggested that through careful design, these models, aimed at children, as well as young athletes, can (i) encourage play and facilitate physical activity and motor learning in children of different ages, providing them with the foundational skills needed for leading active lives; and (ii), develop young athletes in elite sports programmes in an ethical, enriching and supportive manner.

Through this text, scientists, academics and practitioners in the sub-disciplines of motor learning and motor development, physical education, sports pedagogy and physical activity and exercise domains will better understand how to design programmes that encourage play and thereby develop the movement skills, self-regulating capacities, motivation and proficiency of people, so that they can move skilfully, effectively and efficiently while negotiating changes throughout the human lifespan.

James Rudd is a senior lecturer in Physical Education at Liverpool John Moores University, UK; his research interests are in the areas of pedagogy, child development and motor learning.

Ian Renshaw is an associate professor of Human Movement and Sports Science at Queensland University of Technology, Australia.

Geert J.P. Savelsbergh is head of the Motor Learning & Performance section of the Amsterdam Movement Sciences & Institute for Brain and Behaviour at the Vrije Universteit, Netherlands.

Jia Yi Chow is currently the Associate Dean, Programme and Student Development, with the Office of Teacher Education (OTE), National Institute of Education (NIE), Nanyang Technological University (NTU), Singapore.

Will Roberts is a senior lecturer in Sport and Exercise Science, and Academic Course Lead for the MSci/BSc in Sport Coaching Science at the University of Gloucestershire, UK.

Daniel Newcombe is a senior lecturer on the Sport, Coaching & PE degree at Oxford Brookes University, UK.

Keith Davids is a professor of Motor Learning in the Sport & Human Performance research group at Sheffield Hallam University, UK (2014 onwards), investigating skill acquisition, expertise and talent development in sport.

NONLINEAR PEDAGOGY AND THE ATHLETICS SKILLS MODEL

The Importance of Play in Supporting Physical Literacy

Edited by James Rudd, Ian Renshaw,
Geert J.P. Savelsbergh, Jia Yi Chow, Will Roberts,
Daniel Newcombe and Keith Davids

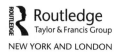
Routledge
Taylor & Francis Group

NEW YORK AND LONDON

First published 2021
by Routledge
52 Vanderbilt Avenue, New York, NY 10017

and by Routledge
2 Park Square, Milton Park, Abingdon, Oxon, OX14 4RN

Routledge is an imprint of the Taylor & Francis Group, an informa business

Library of Congress Cataloging-in-Publication Data
A catalog record for this title has been requested

ISBN: 978-0-367-45794-5 (hbk)
ISBN: 978-0-367-89461-0 (pbk)
ISBN: 978-1-003-02537-5 (ebk)

Typeset in Bembo
by KnowledgeWorks Global Ltd.

Visit the eResources: www.routledge.com/9780367894610

CONTENTS

LIST OF FIGURES

LIST OF TABLES

ABOUT THE AUTHORS

James Rudd is a senior lecturer in Physical Education at Liverpool John Moores University; his research interests are in the areas of pedagogy, child development and motor learning. James explores these areas largely guided by Ecological Dynamics; a transdisciplinary theoretical framework for understanding physical literacy integrating ideas from ecological psychology, constraints on dynamical systems, the complexity sciences and anthropology.

James has over 15 years' experience of working with schools and teachers in the UK and Australia his current area of research is helping develop high-quality physical education curriculums to support physical literacy. James is the lead author of Nonlinear pedagogy and the athletics skills model: the importance of play in supporting physical literacy.

Keith Davids is currently a professor of Motor Learning in the Sport & Human Performance research group at Sheffield Hallam University, UK (2014 onwards), investigating skill acquisition, expertise and talent development in sport. His research is underpinned by the theoretical framework of Ecological Dynamics, examining application of key concepts to learning design and practice organisation in sport, exercise and physical activity.

He has over 30 years' experience of teaching and conducting research with collaborators in UK, Portugal, France, Australia, Germany, New Zealand, Finland, Norway and Sweden in related fields like Sports Science, Psychology, Behavioural Neuroscience, Physical Education and Human Movement Science. He has held/holds research positions in the UK (Manchester Metropolitan University: 1991-2003), Finland (University of Jyvaskyla, Finnish Distinguished Professor: 2012-2016), New Zealand (University of Otago: 2003-2007), Australia (Queensland University of Technology: 2006-2014) and Norway (2020-22: Norwegian Sports Science University (Trondheim), Adjunct Research Professor).

His applied scientific research has been conducted in collaboration with international sports organisations and national Institutes of Sport in Australia (AIS), New Zealand (NZSI), and England (EIS), as well as KIHU (Finnish Olympic Research Committee) and PESTA (Physical Education and Sports Teachers Association, Singapore).

Ian Renshaw is an associate professor at Queensland University of Technology, Brisbane, Australia. Ian has co-authored a number of books, notably Nonlinear Pedagogy with Jia-Yi Chow, Keith Davids and Chris Button, and the Foundation text for the book series Routledge Studies in Constraints-Based Methodologies in Sport; Sport Coaching, Training and Performance: Principles of Constraints-Based Practice. London: Routledge (Renshaw, I., Davids, K.D., Roberts, W., & Newcombe, D. (2019) and A Constraints-Led Approach to Golf Coaching with Peter Arnott and Graeme McDowall. Ian has worked in Higher Education in the UK, New Zealand and Australia, specialising in Skill Acquisition, Motor Control and Learning, Sports Coaching and Games Teaching. Ian's research focus is on applying Ecological Dynamics to sport and education settings. Ian has worked as a skill acquisition advisor to numerous elite sports teams and state and national bodies across the world to support coach education.

Jia Yi Chow is currently the Associate Dean, Programme and Student Development, with the Office of Teacher Education (OTE), National Institute of Education (NIE), Nanyang Technological University (NTU), Singapore. He is a teacher by training and taught for a few years in a Singapore school before returning to Physical Education and Sports Science (PESS) Academic Group as a lecturer. Jia Yi undertook further postgraduate study and obtained his PhD in the area of Motor Control and Learning with the University of Otago, New Zealand from an Overseas Graduate Scholarship (OGS) awarded by NIE. His research interests include examining multi-articular coordination from a Dynamical Systems Theoretical perspective, visual perception in sports expertise and in a pedagogical approach (Nonlinear Pedagogy) where key pedagogical principles underpinned by representative learning design, manipulation of task constraints, functional variability, relevant focus of attention and task simplification can support nonlinearity in learning. He works closely with international collaborators in New Zealand, France, Australia, UK, Finland and Portugal. Jia Yi also has strong working relations with the Ministry of Education (Singapore), Sport Singapore and National Youth Sports Institute (Singapore). For his excellence in teaching, Jia Yi was awarded the Nanyang Education Award (College) and inducted as a Fellow to the NTU Teaching Excellence Academy in 2018. He was also awarded the Nanyang Education Award (University, Gold Medal) and was accorded the NTU Educator of the Year in 2019.

Geert J.P. Savelsbergh is head of the Motor Learning & Performance section of the Amsterdam Movement Sciences & Institute for Brain and Behaviour at the Vrije Universiteit, Amsterdam. Since 2014 he is the Scientific Director of Performance for the Amsterdam Institute for Sport Science (AISS) and occupies a position as Professor of Talent Development at the Amsterdam University of Applied Science. Savelsbergh conducts fundamental and applied research and his research interest lies in the field of visual regulation of human movement. From this perception-action paradigm, fundamental concepts like anticipation and pattern recognition are applied in the sports context in order to contribute to talent recognition and development. He has published over 220 peer-reviewed scientific articles, co-supervised 30 PhD projects and currently supervises 22 PhD projects in the Netherlands, Brazil, China, Germany and South Africa. Together with René Wormhoudt, Savelsbergh is the founder of the Athletic Skills Model for optimal talent development (ASM). ASM collaborates at national level with the cities of Amsterdam and Almere, various sports associations and with various football clubs in the Dutch Premier League.

In the international field, several ASM partnerships have been started in Brazil, England and Japan.

Will Roberts is a senior lecturer in Sport and Exercise Science, and Academic Course Lead for the MSci/BSc in Sport Coaching Science at the University of Gloucestershire. He is a series editor for the Routledge Studies in Constraints-Based Methodologies with Keith Davids, Ian Renshaw and Danny Newcombe. Current research and practice coheres around the application of nonlinear pedagogy and a constraints-based approaches to movement science in elite sport and developmental pathways. He is a co-creator of the Boing project which promotes physical literacy through active play. Will works with a variety of organisations to support the development of learner-centred pedagogies that promote autonomy and decision making of individuals. He is a visiting researcher at Oxford Brookes University, where he is also recognised as a teaching fellow for excellence in developing students and coaches to adopt a nonlinear pedagogical approach to practice.

Daniel Newcombe is a senior lecturer on the Sport, Coaching & PE degree at Oxford Brookes University, UK. Daniel has worked in higher education for 10 years and has been teaching and researching coaching science since his move to Oxford Brookes 8 years ago. Alongside his role at Oxford Brookes Daniel is an international and domestic national league hockey coach. He has been the assistant coach for the Men's Welsh National Team for the past 10 years in addition to his current role as Head Coach of Reading Hockey Club near London. Currently embarking on a PhD which aims to explore the provision of and Environment Design Framework (EDF) to bridge the theory to practice gap for coaches who are engaged in skill development. The EDF is provided to scaffold coaches through the often complex and messy practice design process. Daniel has extensive experience working with coaches across many domains and is currently working with The Premier League, Great Britain Hockey, English Institute of Sport, England & Wales Cricket Board, Welsh Rugby Union & the Lawn Tennis Association.

SECTION I

Theoretical Positioning of Physical Literacy

Section 1: Introduction

Physical literacy is not new, nor indeed is it a well-understood term. The main aims of this book are to revisit the original intentions behind the term physical literacy and explore its links with contemporary models of performance and learning in physical activity and sport. Whilst the concept of physical literacy has thrived throughout academic discourse and educational policy across the globe, the original intentions behind the term physical literacy have become obscured (Bailey, 2020). Margaret Whitehead set out the idea of physical literacy at a conference in Australia in 1993, arguing that in order to support ongoing physical activity, and ensure the healthy development of children, we need to ensure that their movement experiences are meaningful. She expressed concern that children's play opportunities were being diminished and that the activities available to young people were too often over-organised, structured and professionalised, that is, led (coached, instructed, taught) by adults with a performance agenda. Whitehead believed that this untimely professionalisation of children's play activities diminished, or removed, the meaning of the physical activity experience and, with it, the chances of children engaging in a lifetime of physical activity. The authors of this book embrace the concept of physical literacy. We are, of course, not the first to do so, since academic discussion on this topic has flourished over the last two decades (see Figure 0.1).

It is disappointing that this long-running discourse has not led to more innovative methods of creating meaningful play and movement experiences for children through, for example, better pedagogical design, infrastructure or social interaction, or more engagement and exploration of the child's voice to understand what meaningful movement experiences might be for them. Instead, the literature is full of endless academic debate over the interpretation of what physical literacy is and how it should be defined. Indeed, Whitehead herself has changed her definition of physical literacy multiple times since the original introduction in 2001 (see Table 0.1).

Notwithstanding these shortcomings, the academic literature has been influential, leading to the integration of physical literacy into policy across the globe, including the United Nations Educational, Scientific and Cultural Organisation International Charter of

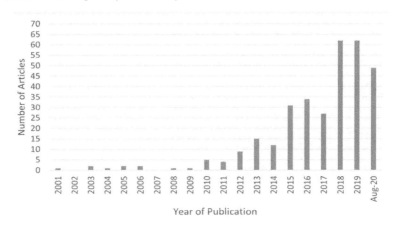

FIGURE 0.1 Physical literacy publications by year of publication from 2001 to 2020

Physical Education, Physical Activity and Sport. As we enter the 2020s, the promises made by academics, and reflected in policy documents, are starting to be questioned as governments are seen to be failing to deliver on their pledges to engage millennials. Generation Z is no more active or healthy than their predecessors, Generations X and Y, and indeed evidence suggests a further decline. The question that we are left with is: Has the prioritisation and adoption of physical literacy been nothing more than a vogue concept lacking in conceptual substance and depth which is destined to fall out of fashion to be replaced by something else that is shiny and new?

This book is a collaboration between seven academics within the field of human movement and sport sciences (motor development, motor learning, pedagogical design and practitioner education). Together, we revisit the nature of physical literacy – a term which was used to describe the movement quality of tribes indigenous to America in 1884 – and we examine physical literacy through the lens of the contemporary theory of Ecological

TABLE 0.1 Revisions of Whitehead's physical literacy definitions between 2001 and 2017

2001	The characteristics of a physically literate individual are that the person moves with poise, economy and confidence in a wide variety of physically challenging situations. In addition, the individual is perceptive in reading all aspects of the physical environment, anticipating movement needs or possibilities and responding appropriately to these, with intelligence and imagination. Physical literacy requires a holistic engagement that encompasses physical capacities embedded in perception, experience, memory, anticipation and decision-making (Whitehead, 2001, p. 136).
2007	The motivation, confidence, physical competence, understanding and knowledge to maintain physical activity at an individually appropriate level, throughout life course(Whitehead, 2007, p. 2).
2010	As appropriate to each individual endowment, physical literacy can be described as the motivation, confidence, physical competence, knowledge and understanding to maintain physical activity throughout the life course (Whitehead, 2010, p. 11).
2013	The motivation, confidence, physical competence, knowledge and understanding to value and take responsibility for maintaining purposeful physical pursuits/activities throughout the life course (Whitehead, 2013, p. 29).
2017	The motivation, confidence, physical competence, knowledge and understanding to value and engage in physical activity for life (IPLA, 2017).

Dynamics which is a transdisciplinary space that blends ideas from ecological psychology, constraints on dynamical systems, the complexity sciences, social anthropology and evolutionary biology. In Section 1, we seek to understand why the concept of physical literacy is still needed today and explore physical literacy from two different scales of analysis: at an individual level and at a community level. In Chapter 1, we explore the scale of the socio-cultural constraints that we faced in the 2020s and seek to understand why current physical activity interventions and traditional pedagogical delivery models are inadequate in developing meaningful movement experiences for children. In Chapter 2, we consider the hunter-gatherer origins of physical literacy as well as exploring Whitehead's original definition of physical literacy. Moving beyond this, we introduce three key principles to understand physical literacy: wayfinding, value and meaning and functional movement skills when conceived through an Ecological Dynamics framework. In Chapter 3, we again explore physical literacy from an Ecological Dynamics rational, focusing on the analytic scale at the higher community level and observe how local-global self-organisation tendencies supporting physical literacy to thrive through spontaneous play in the most unexpected places.

In Section 2 our examination of physical literacy moves beyond the current academic discourse as we begin to explore how we might operationalise this concept to create meaningful movement experiences for learners (children, youth and elite athletes, and recreational sportsmen and women across the lifespan). This may seem like a bold ambition; however, we are enabled to make this leap because, whilst each individual is on their own dynamic and individual journey, the fundamental principles, or mechanisms for how we learn to move, are the same for everyone, regardless of performance levels and needs. In Chapter 4 we explore how motor learning theory has influenced pedagogical approaches right across the sporting landscape. Our aim in this chapter is, through the introduction of a Constraints-Led Approach (CLA) and representative co-design, to offer a contemporary approach which positions the learner at the core of the educational experience within physical education, youth sport and high-performance sport. In Chapter 5 we introduce a powerful pedagogical framework called Nonlinear Pedagogy (NLP) and show how adopting this approach can enable practitioners to reevaluate how they plan and design sessions, activities and lessons to support the learner on their physical literacy journey. In Chapter 6 we continue to explore contemporary approaches as we consider the concepts of practitioners as *Environment Architects* and Environment Design Principles (EDP) and explore how these might be used to support physical literacy. In Chapter 7 we introduce the Athletics Skills Model (ASM), which has been implemented successfully across football academies in the Netherlands and is being introduced into the United Kingdom to support the physical literacy of current and future generations.

In Section 3, Chapter 8, we consider how physical literacy can be measured and suggest how an ecological conceptualisation can help unpick the complexity of measuring something that is, in essence, a process. The final chapter in Section 3 provides a summary of what has been covered and explores possibilities for practice to support physical literacy. Section 4, the final section of this book provides series of practical case studies from physical education to high-performance sport where researchers are beginning to explore new avenues of research to understand physical literacy through an Ecological Dynamics rationale.

1

TIME FOR A RETHINK

Why a New Approach to Physical Literacy Is Needed

Keith Davids and James Rudd

1.1 Introduction

Play is considered to be essential for optimal child development (Ginsburg, 2007). The United Nations High Commission for Human Rights states that play is a right of every child, and yet, opportunities for children to play have diminished. Whitehead was not the only academic back in the early 1990s who was concerned with children's declining opportunities for play and a lack of meaningful movement experiences that were not under the guidance of adults. In 1991, Kaplan predicted that, in the year 2000, the child would need adults to defend their right to play, for society would evolve to provide children with less time to play and increasingly value 'more structure, more work and more adult-directed activity, even for young children (p. 398)'. Kaplan went on to state:

> The child in the year 2000 will be subjected to greater pressures towards beginning academic work early and will be asked to submit more and more to adult-led activities. It is doubtful that television time will be reduced [this was prescient even though the emergence of the smart phone, PC and associated online games were not on Kaplan's radar]. The child may thus have less opportunity to play and less opportunity to direct his or her own play. (p. 398).

Today, we see evidence all around us that confirms Kaplan's prediction, such as the significant decline in children's walking or cycling to school over the past 30 years, which was nearly 50% in the 1970s but had declined to 13% by 2009 in the United States, with similar downward trends across the globe (e.g., Canada, Switzerland, the United Kingdom, Australia and New Zealand). Equally, there has been a shift with children's top ten preferred play spaces transitioning from outdoors to indoors between 1950 and 2000 (Active Healthy Kids, 2014). Whilst the extent and exact reasons for this may be more complex than Kaplan imagined, the explanation he put forward was certainly on the money.

Notwithstanding, the benefits and importance of play are well understood today as shown by a clinical report produced by the American Academy of Paediatrics (AAP) (White et al., 2018) which discusses the 'power of play' to transform children's lives by helping them to combat stressors of modern life and enhance their capacity for learning. The AAP report committee advocates that general practitioners should be empowered to prescribe play activities for children in need of psychological, mental, physical, intellectual and social enrichment (Yogman et al., 2018). Going further, movements like the US Coalition for Play (https://usplaycoalition.org/) promote the health, well-being and social benefits of inter-generational opportunities for play throughout the life course, recognising it as a vital activity for healthy development and the long-term functioning of humans.

A key challenge internationally is that across large swathes of modern society play is seen as a secondary activity that resides behind formalised programmes of directed learning. In the case of the latter, very young children are subjected to educational testing which serves to add pressure on parents and teachers to prepare children to pass tests, often at the expense of opportunities for play and for learning to learn. This 'test-prescribe-test' approach to education was exemplified in 2018, when the UK government brought in universal testing for children at the age of 4 years, upon entering formal education in schools. Another issue is that, as more parents work, children often have less 'down-time' in play spaces, at or near their home, because they are placed in pre- and after- school care. For those who do have the time and freedom to play, the spaces to engage in non-formalised play have often been reduced as land is bought up for development (https//www.theguardian.com/society/2019/jun/02/tory-cuts-force-sale-710-local-football-pitches).

As a brief aside, it is worth noting that an unexpected shift in the levels of children's play was observed in local parks during the UK government's COVID-19 lockdown between March and July 2020. Parks that were generally empty around 4–5 pm each evening were now teeming with children and their parents playing games or riding bikes. Whether these play opportunities were solely due to parents working from home or because organised sports programmes had been cancelled is moot. But what is interesting is that the desire to engage in spontaneously organised, inter-generational play activities re-emerged rapidly when the opportunity arose. These opportunities for experiencing self-regulation in dynamic activity environments like games, playscapes, sports contexts and even urban settings like streets and gardens are at the heart of the enrichment of an individual's physical literacy.

1.2 Physical Literacy and Play

Play is an excellent vehicle to develop physical literacy, as it is through play that children gain psychological, emotional and physical capacities. During play, children acquire a broad range of movement skills, they learn to read (perceive information) and interact with their environment (self-regulate their decision-making and actions). We propose that the emergent tendency to (re)engage in spontaneous, imaginative physical activities is dependent on the level of children's functional capacities; for example, their perceptual-cognitive, physical and social abilities, which are needed to underpin an individual's engagement in play. In most societies, children are not developing these skills. It could be said that 'play begets play', in the sense that individuals taking opportunities to engage in spontaneous, meaningful, imaginative and purposeful play experiences can become more attuned to these opportunities throughout childhood, thus reinforcing their ongoing physical literacy journey. We also suggest that, at a fundamental level, play will have consequences for keeping children safe through self-regulation in everyday environments. This is because everyday interactions with environments involve decision-making, problem-solving and (re)organising movements. Examples include avoiding an approaching motor vehicle, negotiating the waves at the beach and climbing over steep and uneven terrains. These potentially lifesaving activities are synonymous with capabilities developed during play such as jumping over a puddle or a kerb in the street or intercepting a ball at full stretch in the playground or on the sports field (Rudd et al., 2020).

Individuals who have enjoyed rich and varied play experiences throughout their childhood can be considered to have embarked upon a physical literacy journey that will equip them to thrive within, and across, varied movement contexts over their lifespan. In modern societies, this is not a path that a significant proportion of today's children are steadily traversing along. Sadly, across the globe, most children do not have sufficient opportunities to engage in play. Instead, we are observing that physical activity is progressively declining whilst sedentary behaviour increases, typically from the age of school entry (Van Hecke et al., 2016; Colley et al., 2017; Pearson et al., 2017). What we do know from contemporary motor learning theories is that this trend can lead to many children of today having poorer movement repertoires than those possessed by their parents and grandparents. Without the development of a broad range of functional movement skills, other integral aspects of physical literacy (physical fitness, perceptual skills to regulate actions and cognitive functions and capacities) which previous generations acquired subconsciously through daily outdoor play activities also fall by the wayside. This deficit has implications for the ability to learn and function in society as an individual's capacities to discover, explore and act upon surrounding information from the environment are diminished (Rudd et al., 2020).

We know that it is a matter of great concern to governments throughout the world that a lack of movement in children's daily lives is likely to impact upon their physical, social and mental development, and that this will potentially shape their lives as they become adults. Research shows that, globally, the scale of the problem related to children's inactivity is vast, with over 1.4 billion adults not meeting current guidelines of 60 minutes of physical activity per day (Guthold et al., 2018), leading to more than 5 million premature deaths per annum and an economic burden in excess of £50 billion per annum (Ding et al., 2016). It is worth noting that these statistics are not just confined to countries where a lack of physical activity might be explained by environmental constraints, such as places where it is cold and wet, or where there are long hours of darkness for much of the year. Australia, a country blessed with a warm climate, prides itself on being a healthy nation where sport is an important part of its culture. Yet, current statistics tell a different story as Australian teenagers rank 140th out of 145 in a global table depicting national levels of activity. In the United States of America, it is expected that, by 2030, one in two adults will be obese, the prevalence of obesity will be higher than 50% in 29 states and not below 35% in any state and nearly one in four adults is projected to have morbid obesity (Ward et al., 2019; Rudd et al., 2020).

The prevalence of mobile phones, gaming computers, digital technology and media over the past two decades has also become a threat to activity levels. A recent Ofcom (2020) report (Table 1.1) indicated that the current generation of young people are voracious consumers of technology (so-called 'digital natives'). These technological advances are creating a vastly different (socio-cultural, physical, emotional and psychological) environment for children growing up, compared to that of their parents and grandparents. As a result, children and young people in contemporary societies are often deprived of the opportunities that earlier generations enjoyed for engaging in play activities and gaining

TABLE 1.1 Children's media and technology usage from the ages of 3–11 years (Ofcom, 2020)

	3–4 years old	5–7 years old	8–11 years old
Use a smartphone to go online	20%	27%	49%
Watch TV programmes or films	95%, 12 h 42 min/week	98%, 11 h 6 min/week	99%, 10 h 30 min/week
Play video games for	39%, 4 h 42 min/week	62%, 6 h 18 min/week	79%, 9 h 30 min/week
Play games online	17%	35%	66%

relevant psycho–social, emotional and physical skills needed to enjoy meaningful personal developmental experiences (for more insights see box 1.1).

The challenges to modern societies, of a generation 'raised with intense experiences of screen technology', have taken a toll on people's mental and physical health and well-being. In the United Kingdom, some medical training practitioners have reported students arriving for training as surgeons of the future with deficits in micro-movement skills needed to manipulate instruments with care and precision (https://www.nytimes.com/2019/05/30/well/live/surgeons-hobbies-dexterity.html).

These issues have been the subject of academic research in the fields of physical education, psychology, physical activity and the sub-disciplines of movement science for some time. As noted earlier, to combat rising levels of physical inactivity there have been recommendations in many countries that children and adults should take part in moderate physical activity for a minimum of 60 minutes each day. A key question remains: 60 minutes of what? This lack of clarity has been compounded by the vacuous emphasis on reaching an arbitrary number of 10,000 steps per day to maintain physical activity levels. Clearly focusing on frequency data alone, like minutes of activity or number of steps completed,

---

BOX 1.1: PLAY IN HUNTER GATHERER SOCIETIES

Global capitalism has been around for about 200 years, class stratification (chiefdoms and states) about 5000 years, simple farming and pastoralism about 10,000 years, and hunting and gathering at least hundreds of thousands of years (about 95% or more of human history). Foragers today are not Palaeolithic remnants, nor do they live in a world isolated from global economic forces. But the few remaining hunter-gatherers in the world may provide insights into the value of children's play and the failings of the formal education systems. As we discuss in Chapter 2, in these societies life is very different as children in early and middle childhood spend most of their day learning by playing (Gosso et al., 2005; Konner, 2005). Hunter-gatherer children are active learners who participate in learning by choice and need. This is largely because learning is an ongoing, playful activity not separated from the rest of life. For example, children forage extensively, but this is voluntary and not expected by their parents (Crittenden, 2016).

(https://www.youtube.com/watch?v=drJNlGOo0lI&feature=emb_title)

The future is, however, bleak for these societies and very few still exist. Sadly, with their demise, we will lose sight of rich concepts which help us to understand how children learn through wayfinding.

is not providing functional movement capacities for individuals to become active and to maintain an active lifestyle. We believe that the answer is to focus upon making play and physical activity more meaningful movement experiences and this is the focus of this book.

1.3 What Do We Mean by Meaningful Movement Experiences?

There is growing evidence that playing outside with other children on sport fields, public spaces, natural habitats and playgrounds can enrich the broad physical and mental development of children and youth (Davids, Brymer & Araújo, 2016). How, we might ask, can this enrichment process occur? In these varying situations, children need to learn to adapt their actions to environmental constraints such as different ambient temperatures, lighting levels, weather conditions and urban environments (such as uneven surfaces, presence of obstacles, varied inclines and lampposts in inconvenient locations). Quick learning is needed to look out for different, smarter, more adaptive behavioural solutions to make decisions, solve problems and perform skills and create enjoyable games. The learning strategies that accompany playing outside in odd-shaped backyards, convenient public spaces and urban environments can have a substantial positive influence on the development of each learner's psychological and physical health and well-being. From this vantage point, quantity and dose-response efforts like the UK-wide global initiatives such as the Daily Mile (https://thedailymile.co.uk/), where children run a mile around their school playground every day, will do very little to enrich the functional skills needed to take up and maintain physical activity in the long term. There is instead a need to reconnect each learner (children, athletes and recreational participants of all ages) to play in nature alongside the development of pedagogical frameworks that will help us to understand how we can facilitate learning opportunities for children to adapt fine and gross movement skills in coordinating actions in a variety of environmental settings, from stable contexts to more dynamic situations.

1.4 Combatting This Problem by Thinking of Ourselves as Landscape Designers

Research that has analysed experiences of previous generations suggests that previously people had significantly more opportunities to engage in a variety of different playscapes pre- and during formal schooling. This observation has been supported by data from motor development tests which, while not flawless, have been instrumental in consistently highlighting decreases in test scores in different cohorts across the decades. For example, over the past few decades, children in Belgium, the United Kingdom, the United States of America, the Netherlands and Australia, amongst other countries, have continually registered lower scores on standardised tests of perceptual-motor skills, compared to previous cohorts (Bardid et al., 2015; Morley et al., 2015; Rudd et al., 2016; Wormhoudt & Savelsbergh, 2018). Rudd et al. (2016) pointed out that these findings are indicative of the impact of many socio-cultural changes shaping people's behaviours at this time, including the marginalisation of physical education in educational curricula globally, fewer opportunities for unstructured play experiences in everyday life and reductions in open space for children and young people to participate in play and active childhood pastimes. The evidence suggests that reduced opportunities for play are impacting children's functional movement capacities, as registered in differences across the cohorts. It is interesting to note that the effects of changing playscape accessibility and design in modern societies have not only had an impact on children's functional movement skills but also on the depth of pedagogical practices that practitioners (coaches, teachers, community workers) employ due to the environments that they are situated in.

The Irene Marsh College of Physical Education (currently home of Liverpool John Moores Physical Education course) dates back to 1900 when Irene Mabel Marsh started a revolution in physical education by demonstrating that girls, as well as boys, should receive instruction in physical education. Since this time, IM Marsh Campus has been at the forefront of physical education and teacher training for over 100 years. For example, IM Marsh's innovative and feminist approach was pivotal through the late 1940s and 1950s, acting as an advocate for the application of Rudolf Laban's work in modern educational dance, games and gymnastics as well developing 'Moving and Growing' (Laban, 1952) and 'Planning the Programme' (Laban, 1953) both of which were published by the Department of Education in England. These texts promoted a curriculum and instructional model called a movement education, which included exploration, repetition, discovery learning, versatility and quality in movement. This model was adopted in the late 1950s and 1960s but declined during the 1970s to be replaced by the introduction of performance-related coaching at a time when traditional linear and cognitive theories of motor learning were the emerging vogue. Figure 1.1 highlights the opportunities that our current generation and local community of Aigburth, Liverpool, UK has lost.

Gill (2007) has lamented the fact that children are growing up in a risk-averse society where unstructured forms of play, interactions with nature and opportunities for adapting to more variable environments are constantly decreasing (see Figure 1.2). These opportunities for unstructured play are needed to enable children and adults to acquire, adapt and maintain the requisite skills and capacities to sustain continued interactions from infancy to old age (Yeh et al., 2016).

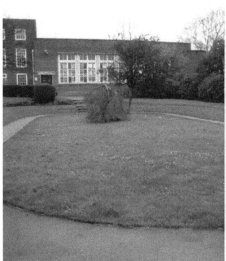 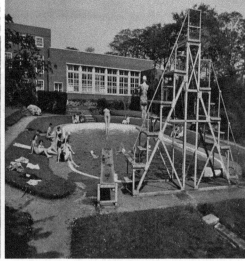

FIGURE 1.1 Irene Mabel Marsh Campus Liverpool John Moores University home of physical education and sport courses (image on the left taken in 2020, image on the right taken in 1950)

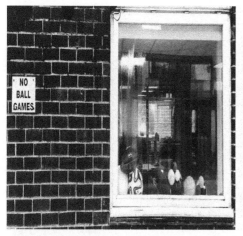
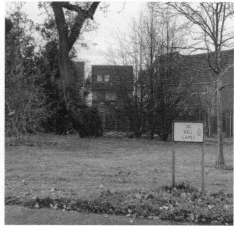

FIGURE 1.2 Common no ball game signs seen in today's society highlighting the risk-averse society

The decline of rich landscapes that afford informal and unstructured play has been accompanied by the rise in modern playscapes that are highly symmetrical and lacking in the variability and challenge needed for children and young people, beyond basic entry-level interactions. Adding more variability and designing asymmetrical playscapes (e.g., changing dimensions, properties like height, depth and shape) can help children to continually adapt their actions and solve movement problems in negotiating the constraints of the play area (Jongeneel, Withagen & Zaal, 2015; see Figures 1.3–1.5).

A major consequence of these reductions in opportunities for unstructured, exploratory play and practice in modern society is the failure to enrich perceptual-motor skills, which act as a foundation for brain development and health (Walsh, 2004), and give children the

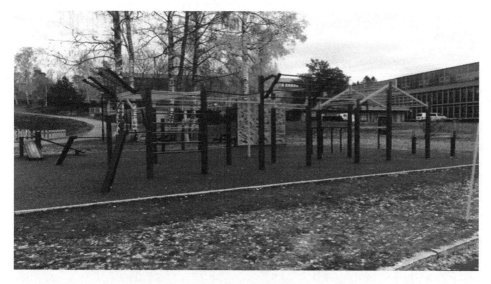

FIGURE 1.3 Example of playground that is largely symmetrical (distance between bars, depth and surface area) therefore affords climbing vertically

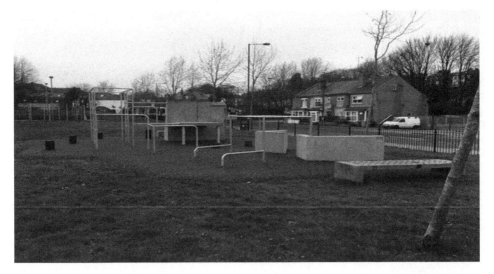

FIGURE 1.4 Example of playground that is asymmetrical (variety of surfaces that differ in height, depth and shape) and therefore affords a wide variety of movement skills to emerge

functional capacities, motivation and confidence needed to learn more specialised skills at a more advanced stage of development. Gibson (1979) referred to these functional characteristics of an individual as 'effectivities' which allow each person to negotiate complex environments. As Wormhoudt and Savelsbergh (2018) explained, this deficit of opportunities for play and practice impacts children's 'physical intelligence', meaning their diminished capacity limits the capability to solve problems through their movements and actions as they negotiate complex performance environments. This deficit can also continue into adulthood, shaping parents' child-rearing practices, and into older ages where individuals may be inhibited from engaging in new movement activities, experiences and sports. Woods et al. (2020) argued that people need physical literacy to find their way confidently

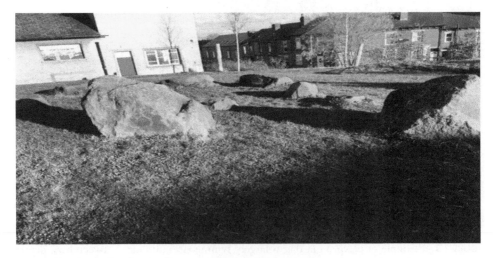

FIGURE 1.5 Example of natural asymmetrical natural playscape

BOX 1.2: KINDERGARTEN IN KYOTO, JAPAN, USING PRINCIPLES OF UNSTRUCTURED PLAY AND LEARNING IN CHILDREN'S DEVELOPMENT

There are some rare, but valuable, examples emerging of educational programmes, which are adult-led, but which retain principles of unstructured play and activity in enriched environments that promote children's learning and development. For example, this kindergarten in Kyoto, Japan, promotes learning in enriched playscapes which have few boundaries which can class them as either indoor or outdoor: (https://www.ted.com/talks/takaharu_tezuka_the_best_kindergarten_you_ve_ever_seen).

Although adults are present, the children are free to explore their environment which is designed in a vast, circular playscape full of opportunities to perceive information and act upon it. These principles include self-regulation during learning, learning through physical activity, having fun and enjoyment and playing independently or in small groups. Evidence shows that some children were tracked over 6 km in an active learning session.

In today's society there is a need more than ever to design landscapes and playscapes which invite, or even require, continuous navigation, and engagement of children in play activities. Arguably, the need for children to develop physical literacy may never have been more important than at this present moment in time, and we will explore this contention further in Chapter 2.

through dynamic and variable performance contexts, by picking up relevant information to guide their decision-making, problem-solving and coordination of actions, highlighting that children of hunter-gatherer societies are far more skilled at this than children growing up in the modern world. There are however pockets of excellent practice all around us in modern society as shown in Box 1.2.

In summary, 'unstructured' children's play-based activities (Roberts, Newcombe & Davids, 2019; Button et al., 2020; Chow et al., 2020) can enrich relevant behaviours including perceiving information, coordinating actions, making decisions, cooperating with others in groups and teams, working to achieve intended actions, solving problems and emotionally regulating behaviours under different conditions in life. It is becoming increasingly apparent that play experiences are vital for human health, well-being and development, for learning and enriching relevant skills and for confidently self-regulating in complex environments. The development of these precious skills and capacities impacts each individual's capability to negotiate dynamic contexts, acquire more advanced functionality through adapting their performance to the environmental demands that they face and to enjoy the psycho–social and physiological benefits of participation in sport and exercise.

1.5 The Problem with Professionalisation of Children and Youth Physical Activity Opportunities

Based on the issues and problems we have discussed in this chapter, there may be a temptation for practitioners, parents and educators to counteract societal and environmental constraints that decrease meaningful play opportunities, by providing children with highly structured, formalised physical activity experiences or specialised sports training programmes. This approach makes good sense when predicated on tenets of a deliberate practice approach to sports training and expertise development, for it has been well publicised that it is considered 'essential' to undertake an average of 10,000 hours of intense, deliberate practice to become expert in a sport (Ericsson, Krampe & Tesch-Römer, 1993). Over the past two decades this has resulted in increased pressure for earlier and earlier specialisation in order to ensure children and young people achieve this target number of hours in deliberate practice. In many countries across the world, it has become a 'trend' to identify, select and train children to participate in sport at younger and younger ages. This belief has created some startling efforts to drive athlete development. For example, in February 2015, the Chinese President Xi Jinping announced a 'football reform plan' to lift China from 82nd place in FIFA's world rankings. This development programme required no less than the country's *babies* being encouraged to grasp the opportunity to develop their talent as footballers (see http://www.bbc.co.uk/sport/0/football/31658273). The 'Evergrande Football School' is a full-time boarding primary and secondary football school with 2,800 students who specialise in football training nearly every day. This programme, costing 2 billion yen, offers extensive facilities, including accommodation, an education building, a training centre, a performance testing laboratory, a conference auditorium and 48 football fields. This example of early specialisation to produce 'talented' footballers underlines our earlier criticism of the treatment of children as 'mini-adults', with increasing professionalisation of children's sport. In 2011, the English Premier League introduced the notion of children in professional club academies maintaining a 'performance clock' to record the number of hours spent in deliberate practice as part of its Elite Player Performance Plan. Some professional clubs in the English Premier League have created an 'elite' squad of under-5-year-old children for the purposes of developing the next generation of talented professional footballers. However, in 2019, the UK Coaching Head of Talent and Performance, Nick Levett, described the approach of some academies, to identify, select and provide such young children with specialised training, as 'madness' (http://trainingground.guru/articles/manchester-city-under-5s-elite-squad-described-as-absolute-madness).

1.5.1 Why Is Early Specialisation Such a Big Problem for Physical Literacy?

A careful analysis of the research on identification and selection of children aged under 5 years as 'talented, elite athletes', suggests that this pathway is not effective because there are challenges in identifying 'talented' or 'gifted' athletes at a very young age (Coutinho et al., 2016). Specifically, early specialisation and dedication to intense training in one sport can lead to problems of physical and psychological health and well-being. In a recent editorial analysis of problems facing children in contemporary societies in the *British Journal of Sports Medicine*, Roetert, Ellenbecker and Kriellaars (2018) identified health and well-being issues emerging from traditional models of sports participation. They considered the main issues to be elitism and over-specialisation at an early age. Previous research by the authors of this book has drawn attention to evidence from the scientific literature on the suboptimality of over-emphasising a one-sided approach to sport specialisation, especially at an inappropriate time (such as at a very early age when children are psychologically, physically and emotionally unready for the rigours of specialised sports training) (Coutinho et al., 2016; Wormhoudt & Savelsbergh, 2018). As we have already pointed out, there are weaknesses of an early specialisation approach which can cause many problems and difficulties for children and young people on such pathways in sports training programmes (Button et al., 2020; Chow et al., 2020).

This approach is aligned with outcomes of a statistical analysis of children by Barth and colleagues (2020) who used advanced machine learning techniques to investigate the importance of coach-led practice in an athlete's main sport and other sports in the achievement of international medals. They found that before the age of 14 years, coach-led activity in a varied range of sports was the most important predictor of international success compared to specialising in just one sport before the age of 14. Taken together, qualitative information on participant insights and the data reported in these statistical analyses provide a useful rationale for enriching learner experiences in play, physical education and sports programmes. They are most useful when considered alongside powerful theoretical concepts and principles of contemporary motor learning approaches such as Ecological Dynamics. Alongside a wealth of other studies (for example captured by Coutinho et al., 2016) perhaps their main value is in raising questions over excessive involvement in specialised coaching in single-sport practice programmes at an early age. This practice has been challenged by pedagogical frameworks such as NLP and the ASM (Chow et al., 2015; Wormhoudt & Savelsbergh, 2018) which we discuss in detail in Chapters 5 and 7. Taken together, the evidence emphasises the need for learners to engage in an extensive range of physical activities and play, both structured and unstructured, which enhances physical literacy of individuals over the life course.

An important message from this book is that specialised practice and training is absolutely necessary to succeed in high-level sports. However, the key issue is to engage in such intense and dedicated programmes at the right time in an individual's development. Typically, specialised training and practice can be most useful after a prolonged period of enrichment through exposure to a diverse range of physical activities and unstructured, as well as some structured, play, games and movement experiences (Bondarchuk, 2008; Wormhoudt & Savelsbergh, 2018; Button et al., 2020; Chow et al., 2020). An essential issue to consider when creating meaningful organised movement experiences concerns how the lesson or session should be structured. A frequent criticism levelled at sport or physical education sessions in, and outside of, the educational system is that, more often than not, the session is delivered as a series of sport techniques, often due to the rigid and inflexible infrastructure of the sporting club or educational institution. The result of this overly structured practice approach leads to a constrained practitioner with little option but to provide a learner with a narrow multi-skills or team sports curriculum (Kirk, 2010). From the learners' perspective, the experience can be prescriptive since they receive constant instructions/corrective feedback for reproducing forms of movements or patterns of play (Chen et al., 2008; Davids et al., 2012). We argue that due to its rigidity and one-size-fits-all focus, this approach fails to support physical literacy. The other issue that we often come across in adult-led sessions is that practice environments are the same week-in week-out, and are focused upon, and emphasise, frequency-based metrics, such as the number of hours spent in practice, the number of repetitions or even the time spent in certain intensity thresholds. Programmes that are based on such metrics are implicated in high dropout rates recorded from development programmes for talented youth athletes in high-performance sports (Côté et al., 2009; Coutinho et al., 2016). However, there are some contemporary pedagogical frameworks which do suggest how the well-documented challenges and problems of early specialisation can be avoided and will support physical literacy.

1.6 Supporting and Developing Physical Literacy: Current Understanding

Based on everything we have discussed up to now, it is perhaps not surprising that today's generation of children is less likely to engage as meaningfully in lifelong physical activity as earlier generations (Barnett et al., 2008; Tester, Ackland & Houghton, 2014; Bardid et al., 2015). In response to this worrying picture of inactivity, the concept of physical literacy has gained in prominence in the fields of physical activity, education, sport, recreation, and public health (Whitehead 2010; Dudley et al., 2017; Edwards et al., 2018). The reasons for this renewed interest in physical literacy may be focused on health and well-being issues, as well as the challenges of developing learners who are confident and motivated to engage in, and maintain interest in, sports and physical activities throughout their life course (see box 1.3 for more information).

BOX 1.3: PHYSICAL LITERACY AROUND THE WORLD

Physical literacy has been formally adopted into the aims of PE curricula across a number of countries (Australian Sports Commission, 2018; PSHE, 2019; Shape America, 2019; Sport New Zealand, 2019; Sport Wales, 2019).

In Canada, physical literacy has been utilised as 'the cornerstone of both participation and excellence in physical activity and sport for all' and it focuses on the physical, affective and cognitive domains. A comprehensive approach has also been adopted in Australia where physical literacy has been integrated into the physical, psychological, social and cognitive domains and has been broken down into 30 elements which are accompanied by a five-step, staged approach for implementation (Sport Australia, 2019). In the United Kingdom, physical literacy has been reduced to a checklist set of capabilities and achievements that every child should achieve (Sport England, Strategy, 2016), whilst in Sweden it informs assessments in physical education.

1.7 An Alternative Solution to Supporting Physical Literacy

In this book, we advocate that children's physical activities should, in many ways, resemble play if we are to develop meaningful movement experiences which can provide a valuable foundation for wayfinding throughout life. This approach encourages play in nature, and carefully designed play experiences that enrich learning opportunities. As a child moves along their physical literacy journey, a diverse range of sport and movement experiences should be sought out that can enrich later specialisation in a sport when athletes are psychologically, emotionally and physically ready for the demands of practice (Wormhoudt & Savelsbergh, 2018; Chow et al., 2020). This book explores the design process by which this might be achieved and offers practitioners insights to enable them to create programmes which support the development of physical literacy in learners.

In the next section, we look at the origins of the concept of physical literacy and review how it is aligned with the enrichment of our functional capacities and behaviours, enabling a meaningful engagement in exercise, physical activity and sport. We introduce an Ecological Dynamics rationale for physical literacy and suggest that this is beneficial to individuals at all levels of performance, including novice, recreational, sub-elite and elite athletes. These benefits are (i) maintaining health and well-being through participation in physical activity and sport; (ii) enriching athleticism and functionality to facilitate movement coordination and skill adaptation and (iii) enhancing the performance of athletes who seek to specialise at the appropriate moment in their development.

References

Active Healthy Kids (2014). Is Sport Enough? The 2014 Active Healthy Kids Australia Report Card on Physical Activity for Children and Young People. Retrieved from https://www.activehealthykidsaustralia.com.au/siteassets/documents/ahka_reportcard_shortform_web.pdf

Australian Sports Commission (2018). Draft Australian physical literacy standard: Explaining the standard. Retrieved from https://research-management.mq.edu.au/ws/portalfiles/portal/83466646/72163645.pdf

Bailey, R. (2020). Defining physical literacy: making sense of a promiscuous concept, Sport in Society. doi:10.1080/17430437.2020.1777104.

Barnett, L. M., Van Beurden, E., Morgan, P. J., Brooks, L. O., Beard, J. R. (December 2008). Does childhood motor skill proficiency predict adolescent fitness? *Medicine & Science in Sports and Exercise*, *40*(12), 2137–2144. doi: 10.1249/MSS.0b013e31818160d3. PMID: 18981934.

Bardid, F., Rudd, J. R., Lenoir, M., Polman, R. & Barnett., L. M. (2015). Cross-cultural comparison of motor competence in children from Australia and Belgium. *Frontiers in Psychology*, *6*. doi:10.3389/fpsyg.2015.00964.

Barth, M., Güllich, A., Raschner, C. & Emrich, E. (2020). The path to international medals: A supervised machine learning approach to explore the impact of coach-led sport-specific and non-specific practice. *PloS One*, *15* (12).

Bondarchuk, A. (2008). *Transfer of training in sports*. Muskegon, MI: Ultimate Athlete Concepts.

Button, C., Seifert, L., Chow, J. Y., Davids, K. & Araujo, D. (2020). *Dynamics of skill acquisition: An ecological dynamics approach*. Champaign, IL: Human Kinetics Publishers.

Chen, A., Martin, R., Ennis, C. D. & Sun, H. (2008). Content specificity of expectancy beliefs and task values in elementary physical education. *Research Quarterly for Exercise and Sport*, *79*(2), 195–208.

Chow, J. Y., Davids, K., Button, C. & Renshaw, I. (2015). *Nonlinear pedagogy in skill acquisition: An introduction*. New York, NY: Routledge.

Chow, J. Y., Davids, K., Renshaw, I. & Rudd, J. (2020). Nonlinear pedagogy. In M. A. Peters & R. Heraud (Eds.), *Encyclopedia of educational innovation* (pp. 1–7). Singapore: Springer.

Colley, R. C., Carson, V., Garriguet, D., Janssen, I., Roberts, K. C. & Tremblay, M. S. (2017). Physical activity of Canadian children and youth, 2007 to 2015. *Health Reports, 28*(10), 8–16.

Coutinho, P., Mesquita, I., Davids, K., Fonseca, A. M. & Côté, J. (2016). How structured and unstructured sport activities aid the development of expertise in volleyball players. *Psychology of Sport and Exercise*, *25*, 51–59.

Côté, J., Lidor, R., Hackfort, D. (2009). ISSP position stand: to sample or to specialize? Seven postulates about youth sport activities that lead to continued participation and elite performance. *International Journal of Sport and Exercise Psychology*, *9*, 7–17.

Crittenden, A. N. (2016). Children's foraging and play among the Hadza. Origins and implications of the evolution of childhood (pp. 155–172). Albuquerque: University of New Mexico Press.

Davids, K., Araujo, D. & Brymer, E. (2016). Designing affordances for physical activity: An ecological dynamics perspective. *Sports Medicine*, *46*, 933–938. doi:10.1007/s40279-016-0511-3.

Davids, K., Araújo, D., Hristovski, R., Passos, P. & Chow, J. Y. (2012). Ecological dynamics and motor learning design in sport. In N. J. Hodges & A. M. Williams (Eds.), *Skill acquisition in sport: Research, theory and practice* (2nd ed., pp. 112–130). London: Routledge.

Ding, D., Lawson, K. D., Kolbe-Alexander, T. L., Finkelstein, E. A., Katzmarzyk, P. T., Van Mechelen, W. & Pratt, M. (2016). The economic burden of physical inactivity: A global analysis of major noncommunicable diseases. *The Lancet*, *388*, 1311–1324. doi:10.1016/S0140-6736(16)30383-X.

Dudley, D., Cairney, J., Wainwright, N., Kriellaars, D. & Mitchell, D. (2017). Critical considerations for physical literacy policy in public health, recreation, sport, and education agencies. *Quest, 69*, 436–452.

Edwards, L. C., Bryant, A. S., Keegan, R. J., Morgan, K., Cooper, S. M. & Jones, A. M. (2018). 'Measuring' physical literacy and related constructs: A systematic review of empirical findings. *Sports Medicine, 48*(3), 659–682.

Ericsson, K. A., Krampe, R. T. & Tesch-Römer, C. (1993). The role of deliberate practice in the acquisition of expert performance. *Psychological Review, 100*, 363.

Gibson, J. J. (1979). *The ecological approach to visual perception.* Boston, MA: Houghton, Mifflin and Company.

Gill, T. (2007). No fear: Growing up in a risk averse society. London, England: Calouste Gulbenkian Foundation..

Ginsburg, K. R. (2007). The importance of play in promoting healthy child development and maintaining strong parent-child bonds. *Pediatrics, 119*(1), 182–191.

Gosso, Y., Otta, E., Morais, M. L. S., Ribeiro, F. J. L. & Bussab, V. S. R. (2005). Play in hunter-gatherer society. In A. D. Pellegrini & P. K. Smith (Eds.), *The nature of play: Great apes and humans* (pp. 213–253). New York, NY: Guilford Press.

Guthold, R., Stevens, G. A., Riley, L. M. & Bull, F. C. (2018). Worldwide trends in insufficient physical activity from 2001 to 2016: A pooled analysis of 358 population-based surveys with 1·9 million participants. *The Lancet Global Health, 6*, 1077–1086. doi: 10.1016/S2214-109X(18)30357-7.

IPLA [International Physical Literacy Association] (2017). IPLA definition. https://www.physical-literacy.org.uk/.

Jongeneel, D., Withagen, R. & Zaal, F. T. (2015). Do children create standardized playgrounds? A study on the gap-crossing affordances of jumping stones. *Journal of Environmental Psychology, 44*, 45–52. doi:10.1016/j.jenvp.2015.09.003.

Kirk, D. (2010). Why research matters: Current status and future trends in physical education pedagogy. *Movimento, 16*(2), 11–43.

Konner, M. (2005). Hunter-gatherer infancy and childhood. In B. Hewlett & M. Lamb (Eds.), *Hunter-gatherer childhoods: Evolutionary developmental and cultural perspectives* (pp. 19–46). New Brunswick, NJ: Translation Publishers.

Laban, R. (1952). The art of movement in the school. *LAMG News Sheet* (8).

Laban, R. (1953). Topological explanations and qualitative aspects. *Unpublished manuscript available from the Laban Archive, National Resource Centre for Dance (University of Surrey).*

Morley, D., Till, K., Ogilvie, P. & Turner, G. (2015). Influences of gender and socioeconomic status on the motor proficiency of children in the UK. *Human Movement Science, 44*, 150–156. doi:10.1076/sesi.15.2.149.30433.

Ofcom. (2020). Children's media and technology usage. Retrieved from https://www.ofcom.org.uk/research-and-data/media-literacy-research/childrens.

Pearson, N., Haycraft, E., Johnston, J. P. & Atkin, A. J. (2017). Sedentary behaviour across the primary-secondary school transition: A systematic review. *Preventive Medicine, 94*, 40–47. doi:10.1016/j.ypmed.2016.11.010.

PSHE Association. (2019). Programme of Study for PSHE Education (Key Stages 1-5). Retrieved from https://www.pshe-association.org.uk/curriculum-and-resources/resources/programme-study-pshe-education-key-stages-1%E2%80%935.

Roberts, W. M., Newcombe, D. J. & Davids, K. (2019). Application of a constraints-led approach to pedagogy in schools: Embarking on a journey to nurture physical literacy in primary physical education. *Physical Education and Sport Pedagogy, 24*(2), 162–175.

Roetert, E. P., Ellenbecker, T. S. & Kriellaars, D. (2018). Physical literacy: Why should we embrace this construct? *British Journal of Sports Medicine, 52*, 1291–1292.

Rudd, J. R., Butson, M. L., Barnett, L. M., Farrow, D., Berry, J. & Polman, R. C. (2016). A holistic measurement model of movement competency in children. *Journal of Sports Sciences, 34*(5), 477–485. doi:10.1080/02640414.2015.1061202.

Rudd, J. R., Pesce, C., Strafford, B. W. & Davids, K. (2020). Physical literacy-a journey of individual enrichment: An ecological dynamics rationale for enhancing performance and physical activity in all. *Frontiers in Psychology*, *11*, 1904. doi:10.3389/fpsyg.2020.01904.

Shape America (2019). Physical Literacy. Retrieved from https://www.shape america.org/events/physicalliteracy.aspx

Sport Australia. (2019). Physical Literacy. Retrieved from https://www.sportaus.gov.au/physical_literacy

Sport England. (2016). New plan to get children active. Retrieved from https://www.sportengland.org/news/government-launch-school-sport-and-activity-action-plan

Sport New Zealand. (2019). Physical literacy approach. Guidance for quality physical activity and sport experiences. Retrieved from https://sport nz.org.nz/about-us/who-we-are/what-were-working-towards/physical-literacy-approach/

Sport Wales. (2019). Physical literacy - A journey through life. Retrieved from http://physicalliteracy.sportwales.org.uk/en/

Tester, G., Ackland, T. R. & Houghton, L. (2014). A 30-year journey of monitoring fitness and skill outcomes in physical education: Lessons learned and a focus on the future. *Advances in Physical Education*, *4*, 127–137. doi: 10.4236/ape.2014.4301.

Van Hecke, L., Loyen, A., Verloigne, M., Van der Ploeg, H. P., Lakerveld, J., Brug, J., De Bourdeaudhuij, I., Ekelund, U., Donnelly, A. & Hendriksen, I. (2016). Variation in population levels of physical activity in European children and adolescents according to cross-European studies: A systematic literature review within DEDIPAC. *International Journal of Behavioral Nutrition and Physical Activity*, *13*, 70. doi:10.1186/s12966-016-0396-4.

Walsh, D. (2004) *Why do they act that way? A survival guide to the adolescent brain for you and your teen*. New York: Free Press.

Ward, Z. J., Bleich, S. N., Cradock, A. L., Barrett, J. L., Giles, C. M., Flax, C., Long, M. W. & Gortmaker, S. L. (2019). Projected US state-level prevalence of adult obesity and severe obesity. *New England Journal of Medicine*, *381*, 2440–2450. doi:10.1056/NEJMsa1909301.

White, P. H., Cooley, W. C., American Academy of Pediatrics & American Academy of Family Physicians. (2018). Supporting the health care transition from adolescence to adulthood in the medical home. *Pediatrics*, *143*(2), e20183610. doi: 10.1542/peds.2018-3610

Whitehead, M. (1993). Physical literacy. Unpublished paper presented at IAPESGW congress, Melbourne, Australia.

Whitehead, M. (2001). The concept of physical literacy. *European Journal of Physical Education*, *6*, 127–138.

Whitehead, M. (2007). Physical literacy: Philosophical considerations in relation to developing a sense of self, universality and propositional knowledge. *Sport, Ethics and Philosophy*, *1*, 281–298. doi:10.1080/17511320701676916.

Whitehead, M. (2010). *Physical literacy: Throughout the lifecourse*. New York: Routledge.

Whitehead, M. (2013). Definition of physical literacy and clarification of related issues. *ICSSPE Bulletin*, *65*, 29–34.

Woods, C. T., McKeown, I., Rothwell, M., Araújo, D., Robertson, S. & Davids, K. (2020). Sport practitioners as sport ecology designers: How ecological dynamics has progressively changed perceptions of skill "Acquisition" in the sporting habitat. *Frontiers in Psychology*, *11*. doi: 10.3389%2Ffpsyg.2020.00654.

Wormhoudt, R. & Savelsbergh, G. J. (2018). Creating adaptive athletes: The athletic skills model for enhancing physical literacy as a foundation for expertise. *Movement & Sport Sciences-Science & Motricité*, *102*, 31–38.

Yeh, H. P., Stone, J. A., Churchill, S. M., Wheat, J. S., Brymer, E. & Davids, K. (2016). Physical, psychological and emotional benefits of green physical activity: An ecological dynamics perspective. *Sports Medicine*, *46*, 947–953. doi:10.1007/s40279-015-0374-z.

Yogman, M., Garner, A., Hutchinson, J., Hirsh-Pasek, K., Golinkoff, R. M. & Committee on Psychosocial Aspects of Child and Family Health. (2018). The power of play: A pediatric role in enhancing development in young children. *Pediatrics*, *142*. doi: 10.1542/peds.2018-2058.

2

UNDERSTANDING THE ECOLOGICAL ROOTS OF PHYSICAL LITERACY AND HOW WE CAN BUILD ON THIS TO MOVE FORWARD

James Rudd

2.1 Prelude

As we discussed in Chapter 1, governments and health and exercise practitioners are struggling with the threats posed by rising physical inactivity levels, potentially leading to worsening outcomes in health, life expectancy and associated high economic costs. Physical literacy has been put forward as a solution to this problem as it is thought that this will create meaningful movement experiences for learners which support ongoing healthy and active lifestyles. However, to date physical literacy has failed to make any real impact as the dominant focus in the physical education literature has been on a hotly contested debate about what physical literacy is, how we should define it and whether we should, or should not, measure it. It is not surprising that in the last year we have seen academic articles published with the titles such as *The fantasmatic logics of physical literacy* (Quennerstedt, McCuaig & Mårdhbeen, 2020) and that physical literacy has been coined as a *promiscuous concept* (Bailey, 2020). The authors of this book are strong advocates of physical literacy and the aim of this chapter is to move beyond the current academic debate and to articulate how practitioners (coaches and teachers) can create meaningful movement experiences that will develop physical literacy. We will explore the transdisciplinary space that blends ideas from ecological psychology, constraints on dynamical systems, the complexity sciences, social anthropology and evolutionary biology. These sciences sit under the umbrella of Ecological Dynamics and in this chapter we will go on a journey to see how Ecological Dynamics can bring clarity to the concept of physical literacy. First, we will travel back to the 19th century to explore why Captain Edward Maguire used the term physical literacy to describe the movement quality of Native American Indians and discover how his perceptions can help us to better understand physical literacy. We will then look at how the theory of Ecological Dynamics offers us a means of developing a comprehensive roadmap which will enable us to begin to conceptualise and operationalise physical literacy.

2.2 Introduction

Physical literacy has been put forward as holding great promise and yet it is not a new concept. One of the earliest documented uses of the term dates back to 1884, when an American, Captain Edward Maguire, used the term to describe the physicality of Native

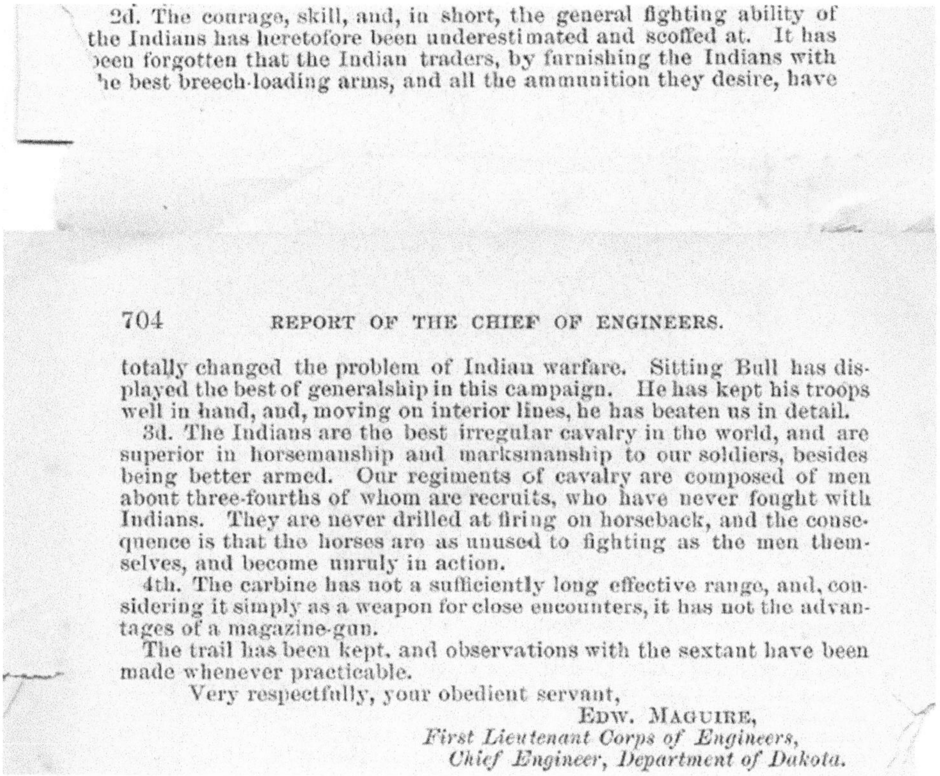

2d. The courage, skill, and, in short, the general fighting ability of the Indians has heretofore been underestimated and scoffed at. It has been forgotten that the Indian traders, by furnishing the Indians with the best breech-loading arms, and all the ammunition they desire, have

704   REPORT OF THE CHIEF OF ENGINEERS.

totally changed the problem of Indian warfare. Sitting Bull has displayed the best of generalship in this campaign. He has kept his troops well in hand, and, moving on interior lines, he has beaten us in detail.

3d. The Indians are the best irregular cavalry in the world, and are superior in horsemanship and marksmanship to our soldiers, besides being better armed. Our regiments of cavalry are composed of men about three-fourths of whom are recruits, who have never fought with Indians. They are never drilled at firing on horseback, and the consequence is that the horses are as unused to fighting as the men themselves, and become unruly in action.

4th. The carbine has not a sufficiently long effective range, and, considering it simply as a weapon for close encounters, it has not the advantages of a magazine-gun.

The trail has been kept, and observations with the sextant have been made whenever practicable.

Very respectfully, your obedient servant,

EDW. MAGUIRE,
First Lieutenant Corps of Engineers,
Chief Engineer, Department of Dakota.

FIGURE 2.1 Lieutenant, Edward Maguire Annual report of the Chief of Engineers

American Indians in his professional notes whilst in the Army Corps of Engineers (Cairney et al., 2019a). As a Lieutenant, Edward Maguire rode with Colonel Custer during the Indian Wars 1874–1876 and was one of the first on the scene after he was killed at the Battle of the Little Big Horn. In the aftermath, he described the physicality and skillfulness of the indigenous fighters and the generalship of Tatanka Yotanka (Sitting Bull) (see extract Figure 2.1 and Figure 2.2 taken from https://hdl.handle.net/2027/umn.31951d00143533a). Later, he used the term physical literacy to capture the movement quality that he observed which he surmised was not taught but was embedded in the very fabric of their hunter-gatherer way of life and the way in which they navigate and 'wayfind' in their world.

2.3 Physical Literacy of Native Americans and Hunter-Gatherer Societies

Hunter-gatherer tribes' epistemology, or knowledge of the world in which they live, is very different to western Cartesian philosophies. For example Native American epistemology is found primarily in philosophies, histories, ceremonies and nature as multiple ways of knowing how to interact with the environment. It is through the close connection with nature, that Native Americans consider knowledge to be acquired, which facilitates a deep connection and knowledge of the environment. This process is partly borne of the need for survival, but it also reflects a deep respect and understanding of the land which is

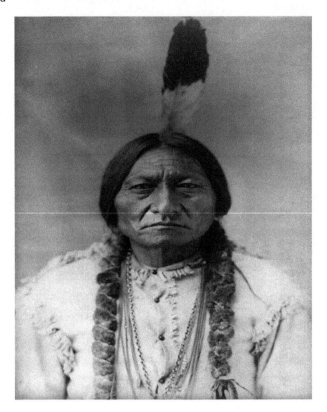

FIGURE 2.2 Tatanka Yotanka (Sitting Bull) 1885

a huge part of their identity and way of life. This is a common factor in the wayfinding of many first peoples across the world and is central to their way of being. They have in common a deep knowledge of the environment as this is their source of understanding how to navigate through the land in order to explore and discover resources, grow and thrive in cooperating groups, to gather medicines and to hunt and forage for food as part of an ecological dependent community. This knowledge of the environment must continuously adapt to the changing landscape as the ecosystem evolves and this is how epistemology is understood to have such strong roots in nature (Ingold, 2000). (https://www.youtube. com/watch?time_continue=3&v=YGRbknDG8Wc&feature=emb_logo)

This way of living in tune with the environment links with the philosophy of phenomenology which purports that something is true when it has been verified by experiences and that this provides explanations which assist in completing tasks. This worldview is dynamic as new experiences alter and add to it. The world is viewed as infinitely complex and so it is impossible to come to a universal understanding of it. Native Americans believe that useful knowledge can only be acquired through individual experience which, whilst subjective, is valid to that space and time. They call this wayfinding, and we would refer to it as the physical literacy journey. The way of interacting with the environment is never fixed and, instead, is carried through generations who continuously revise and add to it. This is passed down through stories, song, feast and dance (see Box 2.1) creating a dynamic web of knowledge shaped by the individual experiences of a community.

BOX 2.1: NATIVE AMERICANS DANCE

Cree, one of the largest Native American tribes, understands the world as an iterative process founded upon interactions between human and non-human things. An illustration of this is when, during dance, tribe members dress in animal skins and feathers, not to cover up, but to unlock the effectivities (Gibson, 1979: skills, predispositions, capacities) of the animal they embody and perceive things they could not in their human form (see Figure 2.3).

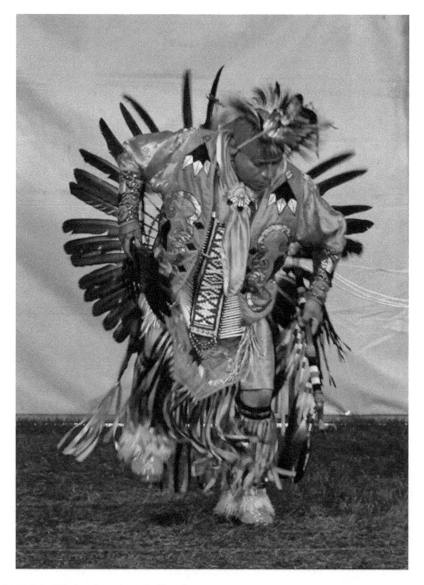

FIGURE 2.3   Native American Indian dancer

Next, we move forward, almost a century, to 1993 when Margaret Whitehead felt the need to revisit and re-formulate the concept of physical literacy. Whitehead believed that play opportunities for children were being reduced and that her role as a physical education teacher was shifting subtly towards curriculums that had a high-level performance agenda focused upon fitness and the drilling of 'sport techniques'. She observed that such curricula and pedagogical approaches put a large proportion of children off physical activity. She promoted the idea that the value of physical activity, beyond the achievement of successful sport performance at international level, was minimal. Whitehead was not alone, as we discussed in Chapter 1, Kaplan had expressed similar concerns and these were also echoed by prominent physical education academics such as Kirk (2010) who described current practice in physical education teaching as that of 'physical education as sport-techniques'. Others, like Shilling (2008), stated that children who experience physical education in schools are now living in an era that will be known as the era of performative sport, where in school physical education and outside of school sport are either overtly or subtly focused on high-level technical performance as the principal focus.

Whitehead's early work on physical literacy emphasised the importance of meaningful movement experiences that embodies a child's cultural history – be that during physical education, or physical activity, and advocated unstructured play. To help her articulate and understand what physical literacy is and how we can support its development in children, she engaged with three philosophical schools of thought that shared similarities with hunter-gatherer and non-western philosophies. These three frameworks are monism, existentialism and phenomenology:

- Monism is the belief that the mind and body are interdependent and indivisible (Whitehead, 2007).
- Existentialism proposes that every person is an individual as a result of their interactions (Whitehead, 2007).
- Phenomenology proposes that the world views of individuals are formed through their experience of these interactions, and suggests that perception, through our embodied nature, forms unique perspectives on how individuals view the world (Whitehead, 2007).

These philosophies can be observed in Whitehead's (2001) definition of physical literacy which is far removed from the elitist picture of physicality and sport specificity currently being promoted in sport, physical activity and physical education (Whitehead, 1993; Shilling, 2008; Kirk, 2010) and moves us towards an embodied description of a meaningful movement experience.

> A physically literate individual moves with poise, economy and confidence in a wide variety of physically challenging situations. The individual is perceptive in 'reading' all aspects of the physical environment, anticipating movement needs or possibilities and responding appropriately to these, with intelligence and imagination. Physical literacy requires a holistic engagement that encompasses physical capacities embedded in perception, experience, memory, anticipation and decision-making.
>
> *Whitehead (2001, p. 131) physical literacy definition*

In this definition, we can see that the monist and existentialism roots reject the dualism of mind and body as being separate entities and instead the world is perceived from the backdrop of the individual's previous interactions. Taking a phenomenological stance, physical literacy means each one of us brings our personal cluster of previous interactions to a situation, and each one of us will perceive the situation from a unique and personal point of view. With the inherent involvement of our embodied capability, in almost every interaction, it follows that our embodied capability will significantly influence our perception. In her work on physical literacy Whitehead (2013) did not, however, explain how this process of enrichment to support the development of physical literacy occurs. Instead, she focused on outcomes, describing certain attributes that a physically literate person exhibits

1. motivation to capitalise on one's movement potential;
2. moving with poise, economy and confidence in different movement settings;
3. being perceptive in reading all aspects of the environment and responding to the possibilities of movement;
4. having an established sense of oneself as an embodied being;
5. having an understanding of the qualities of one's own movement performance as well as the principles of embodied health with respect to basic aspects such as exercise, sleep and nutrition.

Whitehead's decision to describe the universal attributes of physical literacy that one should possess, as a result of continued engagement in physical activities over the life course, moves conceptualisation away from phenomenology, as these attributes are no longer individualised, but are instead aspects that we should aim to develop within all children and adults. This approach diminishes the idea of an embodied individualised physical literacy journey and the underlying phenomenological assumption that it is impossible to compare one person's development with another. This distancing from embodiment and phenomenology continued with further definitional work by Whitehead and the International Physical Literacy Associations (of which Margaret Whitehead is the president) and her view of physical literacy began to reflect modern-day Western philosophies such as the Cartesian worldview (from the French philosopher Réné Descartes), that conceives the mind separate from the body. It should be noted that this opinion is not acknowledged by Whitehead or the International Physical Literacy Association. However, subsequent definitions do, on the face of it, seem to have lost their original phenomenological underpinning, where the individual and the environment are considered as an inseparable holistic system. Physical literacy is now defined as:

> The motivation, confidence, physical competence, knowledge and understanding to value and engage in physical activity for life.
>
> *IPLA (2017)*

These four interrelated constructs: physical, motivation, confidence, knowledge and understanding move physical literacy into a decontextualised arena where we are focusing on the development of the child and their capacities. This definition does not fully take into account the role that the environment and context play within this process. It has been argued that this is a weakness and to address this we will next introduce an Ecological Dynamics rationale which fully integrates a person-environment scale of analysis in conceptualising physical literacy.

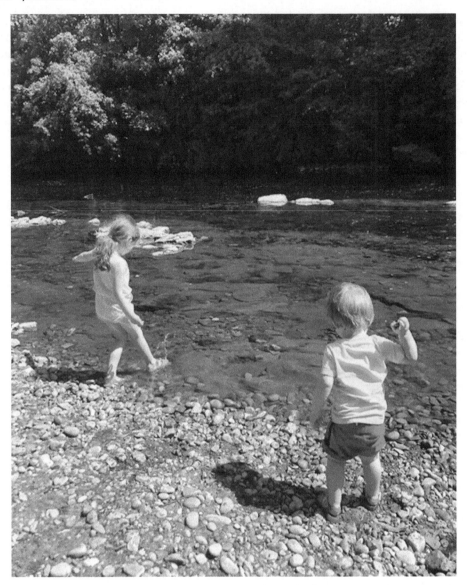

FIGURE 2.4 Two young children playing by a river

2.4 Ecological Dynamics

To begin to appreciate an Ecological Dynamics conceptualisation of physical literacy we will start by exploring Figure 2.4. In this photo we see two young children playing by a river. As parents and practitioners, we recognise that spontaneous playful engagement with such environments is essential for children's development and yet we do not tend to dwell upon this or consider the reasons why play is so important to children's development. In this chapter, we will be exploring why such environments are not only important for children's development but are also essential across the life course. The shallow river creates an invitation, or opportunity, for interaction; the little girl is kicking and splashing the water with her foot whilst her younger brother interacts by throwing a stone into the water. The way they are engaging with the body of water is not driven by a cognitive process, but rather a goodness of fit between the child's effectivities, by this we mean the child's cognitive, emotional and perceptual development and aspects of the environment such as the presence in the water of pebbles, sand or moss, the temperature of the water and other factors such as rain or wind. For each child the goodness of fit is different. The young boy does not have the same effectivities as his sister as he is not so far along his physical literacy journey and has not had as many experiences, and interactions, where skills have been learned and developed. The little boy is cautious and interacts in a way that is safe for him through standing in a bipedal stance to maintain balance (if he was to try to copy his sister and balance on one leg and kick the water he would likely fall over). This is contrary to Cartesian science as this is not a conscious decision, or a process of the mind, but rather the self-regulation of the whole system child/environment. As we will see through the remainder of this chapter physical literacy is a journey of exploration and adaptation of learning in development.

For more than two decades, Ecological Dynamics has been accepted as providing a robust, empirical and theoretically informed view of how we understand performance, learning, skill and development. The theory of Ecological Dynamics explains that movement emerges from the self-organisation of multiple sub-systems within the person, task and environment (Davids, Handford & Williams, 1994; Warren, 2006). According to the Ecological Dynamics framework, intentional actions and movement performance should be conceived as dynamic functional solutions that emerge from the interaction of different constraints (task, individual and environment) as shown in Figure 2.5 (Davids et al., 1994; Seifert et al., 2018; Button et al., 2020). Ecological Dynamics is a combination of several theoretical influences applied to the study of movement coordination and motor learning, including *ecological psychology* (Gibson, 1979), *dynamical systems theory* (Kugler & Turvey, 1987) and the *complex biological systems approach* in *neurobiology and neuroanatomy* (Edelman & Gally, 2001; Price & Friston, 2002). In Table 2.1 we briefly elucidate what each of these theoretical influences bring to an Ecological Dynamics conceptualisation of movement behaviour.

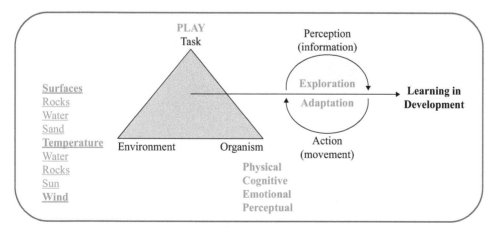

FIGURE 2.5 Exploration and adaptation under constraints

TABLE 2.1 Scientific theories that reside within Ecological Dynamics and help us define physical literacy

Ecological Psychology: We must perceive in order to move, but we also must move in order to perceive (Gibson, 1979, p. 223)	Postulates a constant, cyclical use of information to regulate their movements. As they move it means light is reflected differently off surfaces, creating new visual information that will constrain and regulate action (see Figure 2.6). This is a continual reciprocal process of *exploration* of the environment (Gibson, 1979).
Dynamical Systems Theory Humans can be understood as complex adaptive systems (Davids, Button & Bennett, 2008)	Emphasises the need to understand that complex *adaptive* systems in nature, such as the human body, are constantly changing over different timescales, continually transitioning between states of stability and instability (Davids et al., 1994). For example, in the human body, the close interrelationship between the system parts (bones, joints, limbs, sub-systems) underpins the inherent self-organisation tendencies that constrain the emergence of movement coordination (see Figure 2.7). The potential for continuous interactions between system components gives the whole system a certain amount of nonlinearity which provides inherent adaptability, but also unpredictability in a system which is changing over longer timescales (developing, maturing, ageing).
The complex systems approach in neurobiology and neuroanatomy No one way to perform a motor skill	Highlights the need to understand the movement system as a whole (as well as the larger systems formed with the environment). This conceptualisation signifies that the inherent degeneracy of complex neurobiological systems supports the ability of system elements that are structurally different to perform the same function or yield the same output (Edelman & Gally, 2001). Degeneracy in perceptual-motor systems signifies that children can structurally vary their motor behaviours without compromising function, providing evidence for the adaptive and functional role of coordination pattern variability in order to satisfy interacting constraints (Seifert et al., 2016). For instance, during childhood, we are able to switch between locomotor patterns (e.g. crawling, galloping, walking and climbing) to negotiate various obstacles and reach a target object. System degeneracy implies that there is no one unique stable state of movement organisation needed to satisfy interacting constraints. Several stable performance solutions can emerge, depending on the field of affordances perceived by the child to achieve the task-goal (see Example 2.8).

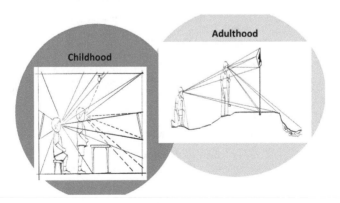

FIGURE 2.6 There is no difference in how a child or adult pick up invariant structure of the environment

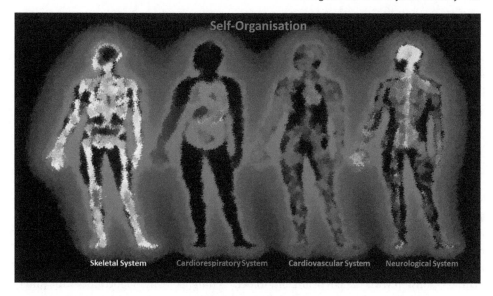

FIGURE 2.7 The human body can best be understood as an complex adaptive system

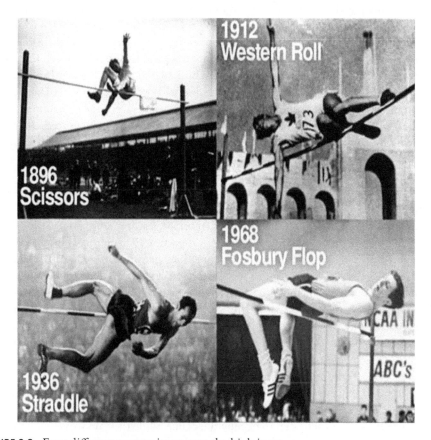

FIGURE 2.8 Four different ways to jump over the high jump

2.5 Conceptualisation of Physical Literacy through Ecological Dynamics

In order to explore an Ecological Dynamics conceptualisation of physical literacy, we need to first set out three key principles that can help us to understand and develop physical literacy in children, these are *Wayfinding, Value and Meaning (Motivation and Intentionality) and Functional Movement Skills.*

2.5.1 Wayfinding – Is Synonymous with Our Individual Physical Literacy Journey

What can we learn from the way that the children of hunter-gatherer communities, such as Native Americans Indians, engage with their environment through wayfinding? In a literal sense, wayfinding is an intentional and self-regulated journey that takes an individual from one region in a landscape to another (Heft, 2013). More directly, to successfully wayfind through uncharted regions of a landscape, individuals need to develop a deep and intimate relationship with the environment, understanding its many opportunities for (inter) action (Ingold, 2000). Hunter-gatherer children have no formalised education and spend all their childhood and teenage years learning through active play and in doing so they develop a deep embeddedness/connection with the environment (Lew-Levy et al., 2018). Mbendjele hunter-gatherer children spend most of their time in playgroups composed of children of different ages which provides an environment for children to learn from each other through continuous interactions and modelling. They climb up high in the trees, using lianas to swing and play 'hunting' by using sticks and leaves. They teach themselves through their observations of adults and other children and through playful imitation of hunting they learn the habits of the two or three hundred different species of mammals and birds and how to track them through engaged interactions with the environment. They also learn countless varieties of roots, tubers, nuts, seeds, fruits and greens in their area are edible and nutritious, when and where to find them, how to dig them, how to extract the edible portions efficiently. The way in which most children live in the 21st century could hardly be more different, and it is interesting to see whether exploring the ecological concept of wayfinding might help us to derive a deeper understanding of our environment, enabling us to interact with it and support a physically literate life.

(https://www.youtube.com/watch?v=15YfjAjumS8&feature=emb_title)

As we have seen, in many countries a high proportion of children do not have sufficient opportunities to play outdoors, unlike previous generations who had freedom to play games in the street, roam around their neighbourhoods and explore local fields and woodlands. Instead, play in modern societies has mainly shifted indoors and has been labelled 'plastic fantastic', that is, adults tend to fill children's early lives with gimmicky toys with narrow functions that don't possess any deep meaning to help them functionally navigate their world. In the light of this, it is hardly surprising that many children possess a functional movement skills repertoire that is more limited than that of their parents and grandparents at the same age (see Figure 2.9).

This decline can partly be explained by the way people live in modern societies. Working parents are often time-poor and prefer to ferry children to and from school by car and organise after school activities to occupy their time while they are working. Perceived safety concerns also limit the time children are allowed to spend playing outdoors. The

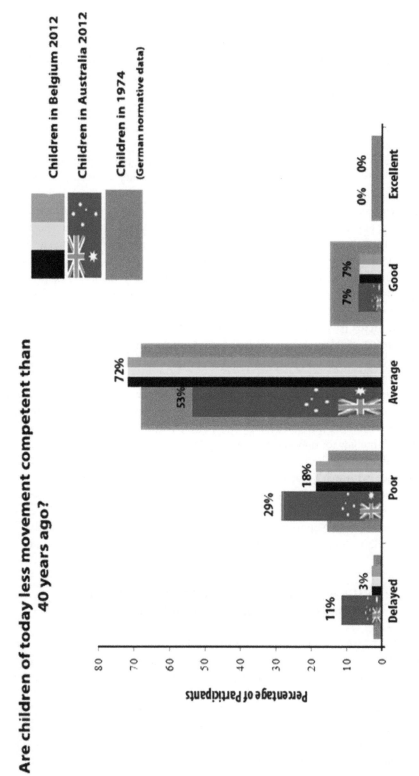

FIGURE 2.9   Levels of movement skill of Australian and Belgium children from 2012 compared to German children of 1974

consequence of this is that children do not have the opportunities to explore their environment and get to know it intimately in the way previous generations have. In this, their lives are diminished, they are less familiar with seasonal changes and how this alters the landscape with foggy mornings or icy pavements. They may not be aware of traffic hazards, and lack familiarity with the street architecture in their neighbourhood, like the high narrow wall you can balance and walk along, or the bollards you can leapfrog over on your way to school, or the steep bank down which you ride your bike in the park and the woods where you can camp at weekends. Clearly, where we can, we should encourage children to explore their local environment, be that inner-city urban areas, the suburbs or rural areas. By exploring and experiencing this first hand they will develop a deep knowledge of the environment. This is a process driven by an individual's capability to detect key and meaningful features of the environment that can be exploited to 'find their way' (Ingold, 2000). Even when required to explore new places and navigate through unfamiliar territory, the child's previous experience will enable them to carefully detect information and utilise environmental features (known as affordances from ecological psychology) to successfully and safely 'find their way' (Ingold, 2000, p. 239). Children will also develop the athletic qualities to quickly reorganise the motor system into relevant coordination patterns that are transferable, as they learn which specific behaviours are more functional than others in different environments, for example moving from a concrete path to muddy terrain or walking along an icy pavement. It is important to reiterate that wayfinding involves *active engagement with the world*, seeking, and being constantly responsive to its invitations for (re)organising actions: whether this action be self-navigating from a known to an unknown destination, or self-navigating through an emergent movement-related problem during play. In both landscapes, it is the individual's *knowledge of* the environment that progressively enables them to skilfully interact with the environment. It is in this way that wayfinding supports ongoing physical literacy.

The physical literacy journey can be considered as a process of entanglement, this means progressively deepening the learner's *knowledge of* the environment (Gibson, 1979), and his or her place within it (Ingold, 2000). The difference between 'knowledge of' and 'knowledge about' is central to the concept of *wayfinding* (Woods et al., 2020). Teachers and coaches often slip into the trap of providing children with knowledge about the environment to support their development (see Box 2.2), for example on the sports field this could be by giving children an overly long and detailed explanation of how a child should play an

---

BOX 2.2: EVIDENCE THAT NATURAL PLAY CAN ENHANCE CHILDREN'S DEVELOPMENT IN MODERN SOCIETY

Dankiw et al. (2020) conducted a systematic review of unstructured nature play on health in early childhood development and found that nature play improved children's levels of physical activity, health-related fitness, motor skills, learning, and social and emotional development. It also showed that nature play showed improvements in cognitive and learning outcomes, including children's levels of attention and concentration, punctuality, settling in class (even after play), constructive play, social play, as well as imaginative and functional play, further reinforcing the importance of natural environments to support children's development.

activity rather than encouraging children to gain knowledge of the activity by experiencing it for themselves. Too often in our society, we provide children with a 'short-cut' to assist them, but ultimately this dampens the development of important skills and 'de-educates their intentions'. Hunter-gatherer communities understand that wayfinding is a journey of self-navigation which is developed through the freedom to explore and interact with their environment and it is from this that we develop value and meaning for physical activity.

2.5.2 Value and Meaning

2.5.2.1 Part 1: Motivation

As we highlighted in Chapter 1, it is common in our society for parents and practitioners to coax children to specialise early in sport techniques and to engage in one specific sport as they believe that this is necessary to gain mastery over both the technical and tactical aspects of the sport. Evidence suggests, however, that early specialisation may actually lead to the emergence of a narrower set of movement skills that will be highly stable, and not easily perturbed, causing inflexibility and lack of adaptability due to the development of highly specialist, rigid functional movement skills that may not transfer across performance environments. This specialisation approach has also been found to be demotivating for children and can cause problems for psychological health and well-being.

In Section 2 of this book, we will be exploring in some detail contemporary pedagogical approaches that have been shown to be effective in providing meaningful movement experiences to help learners acquire skills and maintain a high level of engagement and motivation and hence helping them to value physical activity (Moy, Renshaw & Davids, 2014). To understand motivation and how activities hold value from an Ecological Dynamics conceptualisation, we need to understand that the concept of affordances moves the dial away from the traditional view of motivation as being an internalised process, towards a state which is not necessarily intrinsic, but rather is shared with the environment (Gibson, 2000). James Gibson (1979) considered motivation more broadly as emerging from the individual's engagement with affordances of objects, surfaces, events, or other people in the environment, that may have value and meaning (or not) for each individual. This engagement with affordances can change, depending on experience and a person's needs, a mundane example given by Gibson is needing to post a letter in a postbox. The postbox would solicit the attraction for an individual when they had a letter that needed to be posted, if they lived in an environment where there is a postal system. But the affordance of the postbox would not be soliciting when there is no letter to be posted. The affordance of the postbox is always there and does not change, but the value or meaning (and hence the motivation to use an affordance or not) changes as an individual's needs change. So, in a gymnastics lesson, a high horse with an adjacent crash mat will hold a different value and meaning to children in the lesson than a high horse without a crash mat. The high horse with a crash mat will offer the child the value and meaning to explore a range of different movement solutions in a zone of safe uncertainty. The horse without a crash mat does not hold the same value and meaning and, as a result, the child is unlikely to demonstrate the same level of exploratory behaviour and will appear unmotivated to engage. This may not always be the case of course, for a child who is highly familiar with, and has experience of, the high horse may not feel the need for the safety net of the crash mat for it to provide meaning and value. However, the more experienced child is likely to perceive the affordance of trying to perform a more advanced movement with the crash mat than they would attempt if it was not there. A well-designed activity or environment will therefore hold meaning and value to all children. In such environments each individual is invited to explore an affordance landscape through choosing their own level of difficulty, this will encourage individuals to interact with their immediate environment and modify behaviours in response to changes in body, skills, environment or task (Adolph & Hoch, 2019). From this Ecological Dynamics perspective, physical literacy can, therefore, be understood as the degree to which the properties of each individual and the environmental characteristics match in varying performance contexts over a lifespan. In this way, physical literacy can be conceptualised as the emerging functionality of the fit between an individual and the environment.

2.5.2.2 Part 2 Intentionality

Whilst motivation is the value or meaning one places on an available affordance, intentionality is the discovery of value and meaning during movement. The conceptualisation of intentionality should not be confused with purposiveness, or intent to move, an error which is present in some of Whitehead's attributes such as *motivation to capitalise on one's movement potential* (Merleau-Ponty, 2002; Whitehead, 2013). Operationalising an individual's intentionality, as a form of agency from an Ecological Dynamics conceptualisation of physical literacy, is aligned to being attuned to changing dynamics in the performance context and the pick-up of information to exploit opportunities that emerge.

BOX 2.3: EXAMPLE OF SKILLED INTENTIONALITY

Let us say in a game of soccer, the opposing team is 1-0 up in the final minutes of the game but the opposing team has a player sent off. A child with skilled intentionality will have the confidence, versatility and skills to explore and exploit the new space available to their team. Children who demonstrate intentionality are therefore skilled, versatile and highly adaptable as they are able to exploit self-organisation tendencies (i.e. emergence of behaviours as a consequence of the interactions amongst task and environmental constraints) to regulate their's and others' behaviours, when searching for affordances for a functional movement solution to a problem or task.

Intentionality captures a child's cognition, that is their understanding, planning, (re)organising, problem-solving and decision-making, but it is not limited to cognition as it also encompasses all of our effectivities self-organising under dynamic constraints of task and environment (Davids, Button & Bennett, 2001). This means that the greater the number of exploratory movements there are, will in turn reveal a larger number of affordances perceived for utilisation by the learner (Gibson, 1988). A child's agency in learning and performance is, therefore, expressed through self-regulated exploration of an environment, this means information-gathering in the service of action, which reciprocally guides further perception and actions adaptively in real time. An individual's intentionality is, therefore, intimate and specific to the interacting (personal, task and environmental) constraints of specific performance contexts. This provides both value and meaning through exploration due to the emergence of utilisation of an affordance. A practitioner can interfere with this process if they provide too many constraints on a child's exploration, if they prevent exploration behaviours through repetitive activities that lead to rote practice or if they ask a child to copy the way the practitioner performs the skill. The reason for this is that it prevents exploration and takes away intentionality and, with it, both value and meaning a child can gain from the activity (see Box 2.3).

2.5.3 Functional Movement Skills

Functional Movement Skills are at the heart of our physical literacy conceptualisation of Ecological Dynamics. *Functional Movement Skills* refers to the repertoire of behaviours (cognition, perception and actions) which allow an individual to navigate the environment, interact with others and negotiate tasks to achieve intended goals (Chow et al., 2020). It is the emergence of new functional movement skills that enable new information and, with it, affordances to be realised and new functional movement skills emerge. Another reason that functional movement skills are at the heart of physical literacy is that this is the only way that practitioners can observe and understand children's physical literacy. It is through ongoing observation of children's functional movement skills during play, physical activity and performance settings that we can begin to understand all aspects of a child's physical literacy, both in the value and meaning towards an environment and how deep their knowledge of the environment currently is (for more information see Box 2.4).

BOX 2.4: FUNCTIONAL MOVEMENT SKILLS

Experiences of synergy formation and reformation lead to a greater breadth of stable coordination patterns (known as attractors in dynamical systems theory) to support movement *functionality* which is a fundamental element of physical literacy. The re-shaped repertoire of coordinated movement patterns that emerges through learning and development will increase the likelihood that the individual will become proficient and confident in their own ability to function, and will perform successfully, across multiple sporting environments. This has been coined 'learning in development' by Karen Adolph (Adolph & Hoch, 2019).

2.6 A Possible Future Direction for Physical Literacy

Prior to the recent shift towards the professionalisation of youth sport and physical education, there was a rich discourse in movement education that held central to the idea of the body being an expression of movement, and this led to the development of Laban dance and educational gymnastics where the emphasis was on helping the participant to discover new and more efficient or expressive ways to move. However, this model fell out of favour and was replaced by fitness and skill-based models. It has been suggested that one of the biggest flaws in movement education, that led to its downfall, was its complexity of planning and the difficulty teachers had in articulating a clear pedagogical framework beyond their experiential experience. We will discuss in Chapter 5 how nonlinear

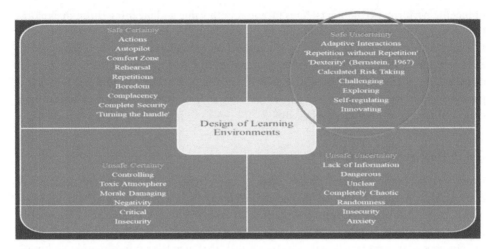

FIGURE 2.10 Design of learning environments aims to design lesson and activities of safe uncertainty

pedagogy (NLP) might provide the new foundation for movement education enabling functional movement solutions to emerge whereby the role of the practitioner is to move the learner outside of their *comfort zone* and into a zone of safe uncertainty. In Figure 2.10, safety refers to learners' beliefs that they are free to explore the environment and discover new ways of interacting with task designs without the fear of negative comments and feedback. Uncertainty refers to increasing information and variability designed into the landscape for learners. In Chapter 10 we will provide two examples showing how NLP and movement education can be combined to support physical literacy.

2.7 Concluding Remarks

In this chapter, we have proposed that physical literacy is an ecological concept, as first revealed by Captain Edward Maguire in 1884. Thanks to contemporary scientific developments in our understanding of Ecological Dynamics and the transdisciplinary framework that resides underneath it, it has been possible for us to outline the four key principles that underpin physical literacy: *Functional Movement Skills, Wayfinding, Motivation and Intentionality*. As we have seen, these are enmeshed together and are indivisible, in the same way that the individual and the environment make an inseparable pair (Gibson, 1979). In the next chapter, we will continue our exploration of physical literacy, but we will view it at a community and collective level, observing in particular how exploitation of local-level global self-organisation tendencies of physical literacy can result in spontaneous play in the most unexpected places. Significantly, these collective self-organisation tendencies for physical activity and play emerge in different socio-cultural contexts, often in spite of national policy, instruction and structured organisation from teachers and community leaders, regardless of built infrastructure or resources.

References

Adolph, K. E. &Hoch, J. E. (2019). Motor development: Embodied, embedded, encultured, and enabling. *Annual Review of Psychology, 70*, 141–164. doi:10.1146/annurev-psych-010418-102836.

Bailey, R. (2020). Defining physical literacy: Making sense of a promiscuous concept. *Sport in Society*. doi:10.1080/17430437.2020.1777104.

Button, C., Seifert, L., Chow, J.Y., Davids, K. & Araujo, D. (2020). *Dynamics of skill acquisition: An ecological dynamics approach*. Champaign, IL: Human Kinetics Publishers.

Cairney, J., Kiez, T., Roetert, E. P. & Kriellaars, D. (2019a). A 20th-century narrative on the origins of the physical literacy construct. *Journal of Teaching in Physical Education, 38*(2), 79–83.

Chow, J.Y., Davids, K., Renshaw, I. & Rudd, J. (2020). Nonlinear pedagogy. In M.A. Peters & R. Heraud (Eds.), *Encyclopedia of educational innovation* (pp. 1–7). Singapore: Springer.

Dankiw, K. A., Tsiros, M. D., Baldock, K. L. & Kumar, S. (2020). The impacts of unstructured nature play on health in early childhood development: A systematic review. *PloS One, 15*(2), e0229006. doi:10.1371/journal.pone.0229006.

Davids, K. W., Button, C. & Bennett, S. J. (2001). Genes, training, and other constraints on individual performance: A role for dynamical systems theory. *Sportscience, 5*, 1–3.

Davids, K. W., Button, C. & Bennett, S. J. (2008). *Dynamics of skill acquisition: A constraints-led approach*. Champaign, IL: Human Kinetics.

Davids, K. W., Handford, C. & Williams, M. (1994). The natural physical alternative to cognitive theories of motor behaviour: An invitation for interdisciplinary research in sports science? *Journal of sports Sciences, 12*, 495–528. doi:10.1080/02640419408732202.

Edelman, G. M. & Gally, J. A. (2001). Degeneracy and complexity in biological systems. *Proceedings of the National Academy of Sciences, 98*(24), 13763–13768.

Friston, K. J. & Price, C. J. (2002). Degeneracy and cognitive anatomy. *Trends in Cognitive Sciences, 6*(10), 416–421.

Gibson, E. J. (1988). Exploratory behavior in the development of perceiving, acting, and the acquiring of knowledge. *Annual Review of Psychology, 39*, 1–42. doi:10.1146/annurev.ps.39.020188.000245.

Gibson, E. J. (2000). Perceptual learning in development: Some basic concepts. *Ecological Psychology, 12*(4), 295–302. doi:10.1207/S15326969ECO1204_04.

Gibson, J. J. (1979). *The ecological approach to visual perception*. Boston, MA, US: Houghton, Mifflin and Company.

Heft, H. (2013). Wayfinding, navigation, and environmental cognition from a naturalist's stance. In D. Waller & L. Nadel (Eds.), Handbook of spatial cognition (pp. 265–294). American Psychological Association. doi:10.1037/13936-015.

Ingold, T. (2000). *The perception of the environment: Essays on livelihood, dwelling and skill*. London: Psychology Press.

Kirk, D. (2010). Why research matters: Current status and future trends in physical education pedagogy. *Movimento, 16*(2), 11–43.

Kugler, P. N. & Turvey, M. T. (1987). *Information, natural law and the assembly of rhythmic movement*. London: Lawrence Erbaum.

Lew-Levy, S., Lavi, N., Reckin, R., Cristóbal-Azkarate, J. & Ellis-Davies, K. (2018). How do hunter-gatherer children learn social and gender norms? A meta-ethnographic review. *Cross-Cultural Research, 52*, 213–255. doi:10.1007/s12110-017-9302-2.

Merleau-Ponty, M. (2002). *Husserl at the limits of phenomenology*. Evanston: Northwestern University Press.

Moy, B., Renshaw, I. & Davids, K. (2014). Variations in acculturation and Australian PETE students' receptiveness to an alternative pedagogical approach to games teaching *Physical Education and Sport Pedagogy, 19*(4), 349–369.

Price, C. J. & Friston, K. J. (2002). Functional imaging studies of neuropsychological patients: Applications and limitations. *Neurocase, 8*(5), 345–354.

Quennerstedt, M., McCuaig, L. & Mårdh, A. (2020). The fantasmatic logics of physical literacy. *Sport, Education and Society*. doi:10.1080/13573322.2020.1791065.

Seifert, L., Komar, J., Araújo, D. & Davids, K. (2016). Neurobiological degeneracy: A key property for functional adaptations of perception and action to constraints. *Neuroscience & Biobehavioral Reviews, 69*, 159–165.

Seifert, L., Papet, V., Strafford, B. W., Gogliani, A. & Davids, K. (2018). Skill transfer, expertise and talent development: An ecological dynamics perspective. *Movement Sport Sciences*, *4*, 39–49.

Shilling, C. (2008). *Changing bodies: Habit, crisis and creativity*. Sage. London

Warren, W. H. (2006). The dynamics of perception and action. *Psychological Review*, *113*, 358. doi:10.1037/0033-295X.113.2.358.

Whitehead, M. (1993). Physical Literacy. Unpublished paper presented at IAPESGW Congress, Melbourne, Australia.

Whitehead, M. (2001). The concept of physical literacy. *European Journal of Physical Education*, *6*, 127–138.

Whitehead, M. (2007). Physical literacy: Philosophical considerations in relation to developing a sense of self, universality and propositional knowledge. *Sport, Ethics and Philosophy*, *1*, 281–298. doi:10.1080/17511320701676916.

Whitehead, M. (2013). Definition of physical literacy and clarification of related issues. *ICSSPE Bulletin*, *65*, 29–34.

Woods, C. T., McKeown, I., Rothwell, M., Araújo, D., Robertson, S. & Davids, K. (2020). Sport practitioners as sport ecology designers: How ecological dynamics has progressively changed perceptions of skill "acquisition" in the sporting habitat. *Frontiers in Psychology*, *11*. doi:10.3389%Fpsyg.2020.00654.

3

WHAT PHYSICAL LITERACY IN THE COMMUNITY CAN TEACH US

Learning Design in Natural Settings

Ian Renshaw and Will Roberts

3.1 Preface

As we have learned from Chapter 2, physical literacy does not emerge in isolation, nor is it a phenomenon that we can 'will' ourselves to develop or self-coach. It is a physical journey through continuous interactions with our surroundings and the communities we live in. In this chapter we will see how individuals, through exploration of their community surroundings, whether urban or rural, will enrich these areas supporting each other's health and well-being through playful endeavours. We highlight that, counterintuitively, investing in elitist structures, organisations and culture will not necessarily result in enrichment of many, and indeed, as has been shown by the professionalisation of youth sport, it can result in the exact opposite as predicted by Whitehead (1993) (see Chapters 1 and 2).

To observe physical literacy in our communities we do not need to look very hard, especially when it comes to children and youth. It is captured in the vernacular terminology of 'jumpers for goalposts', 'la pelada' (exposure to the 'naked environment in play') or 'backyard games' (Coutinho et al., 2016; Uehara et al., 2018; Vaughan, Mallet & Davids, 2019). Many societies and cultures, often in urban areas of high deprivation, have a deep relationship with unstructured activities and backyard games, viewing them as an ideal opportunity for enrichment of their daily lives and an opportunity to signal virtue, showcase, test and hone their skills. In this respect, these culturally entrenched activities allow children, young people and adults to devote many hours to enjoyable, playful activities and learning. Uniquely, the socio-cultural constraints of informal play provide a vehicle for self-regulated practice that are not present in modern-day society, as outlined in Chapter 1. These play settings support individuals' support the principles of physical literacy *functional movement skills, wayfinding, motivation and intentionality* as during play develop unique skills, continuously problem solve, observe and self-regulate their behaviours and coordinate their actions with others. Unstructured play (defined here as activity not organised by an adult or professional) also provides a strong foundation for the physical conditioning that underpins later expertise needed to confidently participate in sport and physical activities at recreational, sub-elite and elite levels (Araújo et al., 2010; Phillips et al., 2010; Renshaw & Chappell, 2010; Cannane, 2011; Renshaw et al., 2012; Coutinho et al., 2016). Research (e.g., Côté, Baker & Abernethy, 2007; Phillips et al., 2010; Renshaw & Chappell, 2010;) has suggested that undertaking inherently enjoyable play-like activities not only provides children with a sound basis for future health and well-being but also offers multiple practice opportunities, needed to succeed at a higher level in sport.

3.2 Introduction

Learning in natural environments by *playing* has taken place for centuries by humans (and animals), and yet there is a need to design learning activities that can take place in natural surroundings. The obvious conclusion to draw from this implication is that there is an opportunity to provide some ideas and guidelines to help practitioners understand how best to facilitate this process because play provides a wonderfully rich context for enhancing physical literacy. Why has learning moved away from less formally organised, structured settings for play and physical activity, and, more generally: Why have we apparently lost the ability to design our own learning contexts and activities in many societies and cultures? In this chapter we will discuss some of the reasons why we believe that play has lost its place as being a valuable foundation for enhancing physical literacy which could support a lifelong engagement with physical activity and sports. We discuss what can be learned from the empirical research across a range of sports, analysing the role of unstructured and unsupervised play in the development of sporting legends. Their insights and perceptions of their experiences may provide some valuable ideas on how to design environments that can encourage future generations to self-organise and adapt their activities through interactions with changing surroundings. Whilst empirical work has revealed the impact of learning across the world in a wide range of sports, including ice hockey (Soberlak & Cote, 2003), volleyball (Coutinho et al., 2016), rugby league (Rothwell, Davids & Stone, 2018), we will focus on the 'world games' of football (soccer) and basketball. We will conclude with some thoughts and ideas that we believe should be considered by those responsible for designing the learning experiences and surroundings of young people, with the goal in promoting a renaissance of play as a key embedded contribution to the quality of the lives of young (and old) people.

Given the well-known importance of play highlighted in previous chapters, Why are we faced with the need to make a case for it? Why do clinical specialists in contemporary societies have to advise medical practitioners to prescribe play for modern children? Adult views on the perceived limitations of play can be understood in the context of the often-heard comment by some teachers, coaches and parents; 's(he) is only playing …'. Such comments betray an underlying devaluation of the activities being undertaken during play, and by implication. Play is not believed to have intrinsic value and meaning for an individual, who needs to be formally 'taught' how to *better* perform a skill or play a game. It is much more relevant for a child to feel the need to learn how to coordinate their activities to achieve an intended task goal through exploration and discovery which can be guided and facilitate by an adult. Similarly, the creativity and imagination demonstrated in pre-practice activities is often seen as 'messing about' and the start of the practice session is framed around 'that was a bit messy; now, it's time to be serious'. These views are not recent and adult-organised, formal sport programmes for juniors have a very long history, particularly in the United States with the Public Schools Athletic League (for boys) being formed in New York City (NYC) as long ago as 1903 (Martens, 1978). From an initial number of around 300 boys, the programme, which was run by educators grew to over 150,000 participants in just 7 years and today millions of boys and girls participate in adult-organised sports all over the world. However, over time, schools lost confidence of, and ultimately control of, junior sport. Their specific concerns revolved around the move away from the lofty, but worthy, ideals of educating young people through sport and towards an over-focus on factors such as 'winning and the associated physical and emotional strain' caused by such a highly competitive approach (Martens, 1978, p. 7). Over time, these problems have only become more pronounced as programmes have become monetised to exploit aspirations of parents and families. In less elitist programmes, a major issue is that the vast majority of 'organised' coaching and teaching of children is being delivered by untrained volunteers who are usually the parents of the children in these important development programmes. Although taking on the role with the best of intentions, the problem is that there is inadequate preparation for these significant roles, with the majority of parents having little understanding of child development (especially psycho-social-emotional enrichment), skill learning and the importance of play. Consequently, time-poor parents are attracted to 'drills' that can have the semblance of 'organised structure', be easily run and require little thought or understanding of transfer to the actual 'sport' being played. In some professional sports, this was seen, probably quite rightly, as a problem and there was a push to introduce more 'expert' coaching into organised talent development programmes. However, the evidence to support the efficacy of such programmes is limited and if a measure of success is determined by 'how many' players graduate from academies to professional level, it could be argued that they are a total failure. For example, a recent analysis of the success of player development academies in Premier League football in England found that the system was extremely unproductive (Calvin, 2017). Only 180 of the 1.5 million players who are playing organised youth football in England at any one time will make it as a Premier League professional. That's a success rate of 0.012%, which Calvin (2017) argued was pretty much equivalent to one's chances of being hit by a meteorite when travelling home from training! As discussed in earlier chapters the obvious lack of productivity of some youth athlete development systems seems to have made the problem of youth development worse by instigating a 'race to the bottom'. Some sports have sought to recruit younger and younger children, with professional football teams in Europe and the United Kingdom, for example, selecting 'talented' children as young as 4 for their player development 'academies'. The problem is not just confined to football. Removing the chance to participate in a wide range of physical activities in order to spend the majority of time developing a sound 'set of basics' is not only a flawed idea but also deprives children of the opportunity to embark on their unique physical literacy journey. It also leads to a focus on a narrow set of skills that are limited to very specific affordances of a target sport limiting self-regulation of effectivities to allow learning in development to take place. By this we mean over time, this narrow, highly specialised approach, will restrict exploration and adaptation and with it both motivation and intentionality to explore the environment will wain and with it the possibility to develop a deep embeddedness/connection with the wider physical activity environments that will support lifelong physical literacy. In short, an environment that leads to attempts to direct learners to conform to adult-defined models of how to play games fails to provide children with the opportunity to develop the emotional and physical capacities that will give them the best chance of achieving expertise. In contrast, play in unstructured environments encourages self-regulation and curiosity, emphasising continuous exploration and enhances movement adaptability that will enable children to thrive across a range of (non-)sporting contexts over their lifespans (see Chapter 2).

A further problem in this seemingly unstoppable move towards early specialisation through structured programmes is that it is not just the so-called 'elite juniors' that are being 'forced' to engage in such programmes, it is becoming the norm for all children, with extensive competitions for children of all abilities. Whilst, on the face of it should be a good thing, the battle between sports to capture children's hearts and bodies is resulting in pressure to focus on one sport from an early age and having a significant impact on children's sporting experiences, with some notable exceptions like New Zealand and Norway. For example, in Australia, Aussie Rules developed 'Auskick', a programme aimed at 4-year-olds, in Canada, Hockey Canada developed the Timbits U7 programme to drill children in the basic skills of ice hockey (https://www.hockeycanada.ca/en-ca/hockey-programs/coaching/under-7). It is important to note that not *all* junior programmes suffer from such problems, indeed some may be well-designed and well-meaning with the needs of the children central to the programme design.

So, how can we judge the relative merits of organised programmes versus play to develop sport skills? Adopting an Ecological Dynamics approach highlights the importance of utilisation and availability of affordances to guide exploratory learning. As highlighted in Chapter 2, affordances are environmental properties that provide opportunities for action for each individual. The landscape of affordances in children's surroundings have always provided opportunities for play and physical literacy was developed intuitively, as 'playing out' was what children did. Consequently, such, manufactured environments such as playgrounds, parks, backyards or natural terrains or even streets and waste ground provide unique environments for children to use to play games and sports. Play or practice environments, therefore, can be assessed in terms of the information present in the landscape of affordances (Rietveld & Kiverstein, 2014) in these environments that can invite actions (Gibson, 1979; Withagen et al., 2012; Withagen, Araújo & De Poel, 2017). Withagen et al. (2017) proposed that these affordances can be conceived of as soliciting invitations for action that can be discovered, explored and exploited, through engagement and interactions. Ultimately, with learning and experience, these continuous interactions with affordances of the environment may enrich an individual's effectivities (Gibson, 1979), improving the capacities, abilities and past experiences that a learner can bring to any performance context. For example, the affordances of the backyards of future cricket stars have been demonstrated to be highly significant in shaping the signature skills they become known for in later years (Cannane, 2011; see Chapter 12, for details). As well as having affordances that shape specific behaviours, these play environments may also have social and cultural affordances that influence the types of behaviours that are undertaken in them. For example, in the section below we discuss how players who frequent the basketball courts in parks in NYC are required to follow specific unwritten 'rules' that have emerged over time, if they wish to participate. Similar emergent 'rules' apply across cultures and are specific to the locales of the individuals who frequent them, whether in street football games in Brazil or rugby league in the United Kingdom, volleyball games in Portugal or backyard cricket games in Australia (Uehara et al., 2018; Rothwell, Davids & Stone, 2019). Significantly, the soliciting affordances of these environments have socio-cultural constraints as they do not sit in isolation from the communities that surround them. Consequently, the behaviours that emerge within them are embedded in the ways of life of their inhabitants. This chapter will discuss how these 'niches' for play act to shape the emergence of foundational physical literacy of participants which are consequential to their sporting journeys.

Adopting an affordance-based perspective removes the need for a dualist debate between 'structured' organised practice versus 'unstructured' play and allows each specific 'practice/play' environment to be judged in terms of the interaction possibilities for the individual. A key part of what any environment offers an individual is how it shapes his or her intentionality and highlights the importance of the culture created in environments as well as its physical properties. As discussed earlier in Chapter 2, motivations are impacted strongly by the intentions of individuals as they aim to meet their own needs in a specific performance context and emphasise how the other individuals (i.e., friends, rivals, adults) can influence intentions. For example, through practice, athletes can learn to utilise specific soliciting affordances that provide resources for development in the performance landscape. But, especially in complex, dynamic environments, this process requires individuals to be allowed to search and explore and choose functional action opportunities suited to their needs. This exploratory and adaptive process may be best suited to learning environments where individuals not only take responsibility for their own learning but are often actively involved in designing that environment by continually adjusting, adding and refining specific rules, for example. This adaptive enrichment of the surrounding niche means that the process of task design by educators, needs to be considered from the perspective of the performer–environment relationship. In these environments, task demands are, generally, well matched to the action capabilities of the performers and adapted dynamically as individuals learn to exploit the landscape of affordances available to them. In contrast, when learning is 'imposed' on young (or older) people there can be temptation to provide prescriptive instructions that overemphasise scripted play, rehearsal and repetition in drills. In such instances, this formal learning approach will restrict and reinforce coupling to very narrow fields within the affordance landscape and limit the individual's opportunities to search the landscape for functional solutions. Play begets play, in the sense that individuals who engage in playful activities can become more and more skilled at designing activities and games that will attune to their own needs to develop a deep knowledge of the environment and hence are more likely to spend significant time engaging in fulfilling and on a skill level, deliberate play type activity (Côté, Baker & Abernethy, 2007). Backyard games are crucial to this aim, and in the next section we discuss some of the empirical research that has explored the developmental histories of expert athletes. Consequently, our aim is to critique the physical and cultural affordances of natural environments and evaluate their contribution to the journeys of elite performers. We will also examine other highly pertinent sources of knowledge, such as documentaries from individuals immersed in the environments or biographies of those who have lived experience of them. Embedding researchers in environments has a long tradition in ecological psychology (see Barker, 1965) and can provide a more in-depth understanding of behaviour episodes typical of the environment of interest by collecting data to find out 'what goes on here? (p. 2)'. Biographies can also be a useful information source as often champions describe their childhood environment and provide pertinent information on the factors underpinning their future success, which may be difficult to tease out from official records. In particular, we will focus upon understanding of the role of informal play opportunities and how they are perceived by athletes and participants to promote wayfinding. As discussed, wayfinding supports the development of the underlying physical literacy to acquire the relevant psycho-social, emotional and physical skills needed to enjoy meaningful developmental experiences that lay the foundations for future expertise (see Chapter 1). We explore perceptions of opportunities to engage in spontaneous, meaningful, imaginative and purposeful play and the self-regulation skills that emerge from those types of experiences. We begin by considering how playgrounds can underpin the development of physical literacy before moving onto highlight how street football in the United Kingdom provides the unstructured play opportunities to support the emergence of talented footballers. We then focus on 'Pelada' (the Brazilian version of street football) and describe how it has had a significant influence on the unique flair and creativity associated with one of the world's great football nations. Finally, we conclude by considering street basketball in New York (NY).

3.3 Built Playgrounds: What Do They, and What Can They, Offer Children to Support Physical Literacy

During the second half of the previous century, many playgrounds were hardly appealing to children and were thus poorly visited (see Jansson, 2010; Solomon, 2005). Jongeneel, Withagen and Zaal (2015) have critiqued playgrounds and noted that a common feature was the obvious symmetry in them, possibly due to the standardised engineering of the distances of jumping stones, bars or the ropes in a climbing net. A potential reason for architects to design standardised playgrounds is the idea they are safer as children can repeat the same movements over and over meaning that they are risk-free and that the skill can be highly practiced and lead to mastery. However, an alternate view understood through the concept of wayfinding is that symmetrical playgrounds may actually be more unsafe as children pay less attention to their footfalls or movements and this potential loss of concentration can lead to injury (Nebelong, 2004). Along the same lines, Nebelong suggests that learning to move in standardised environments is unlikely to prepare children for the 'knobby and asymmetrical forms he are likely to be confronted with outside the playground and throughout life (p. 30). To address the question, are symmetrical or non-symmetrical playgrounds more likely to invite children to play, Jongeneel et al. (2015) asked children to construct their own playground. A group of children with different stepping and jumping capabilities were provided with six identical jumping stones and asked to create their own jumping stone playground and then play in it. The vast majority of the children created a configuration with varying gap widths which were scaled to their (perceived) action capabilities. Clearly, when given a choice, children prefer to play in more asymmetric environments, providing important feedback for playground designers and those interested in promoting physical activity in children (see Figure 3.1).

As we note in Chapter 7 when we discuss the Athletic Skills Model, movement scientists in the Netherlands have considered this question and understand that their environmental interventions (e.g., the layout and features of parks) can have an impact on what behaviour is performed in that setting. Although they do not cause behaviour, the interventions can solicit certain actions and thus make them more likely to occur. We find ourselves acting in definite ways without ever having decided to do so.

As previously mentioned in this chapter, empirical research and evidence from observations have supported the notion that athletes who engage with inherently enjoyable and motivating play-like activities in early development can form an excellent foundation

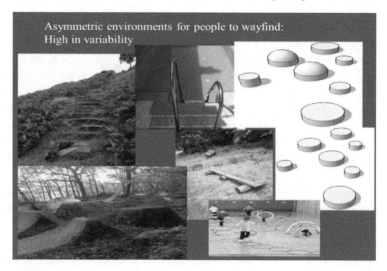

FIGURE 3.1 Playgrounds that are too uniform and 'safe' are unappealing to children. In contrast, children are attracted to play in playgrounds that are interesting and invite challenge and exploration

and impetus to support more specialised training at later stages of their development. In the next section we discuss the notion of 'jumpers for goalposts' in the United Kingdom, and how the modern notion of this, under different constraints, has emerged through activities such as cage football, mixed groups, playing against different ages and so on. In the case of 'jumper for goalposts' we can assert that this type of football has been a 'form of life' (see Rietveld & Kiverstein, 2014) for many young people in the United Kingdom. However, there has seemingly been a decline in the playing of games in the United Kingdom due to the erosion of playing spaces and the formalised and systematic development of coaching, coach education and in particular academy settings for football. As mentioned in Chapter 1, Rudd et al. (2015) assert that these findings are symptomatic of the socio-cultural changes that shape behaviour. The decline in the opportunities to explore the available affordances provided in these less formal settings is eroding some of the best opportunities to promote the emergence of functional decisions, skills and movement. Nevertheless, elite-level footballers continue to report that opportunities to play with older age groups, play on uneven teams, on uneven surfaces and sometimes without a 'proper' ball as the key to their development. Machado et al. (2019, p. 176) support the importance of informal learning for football, stating 'when examining the development process of elite football players, it is useful to highlight the importance of deliberate play'. Consequently, the practice conditions that children are exposed to in early childhood can be seen as fundamental to long-term development, and particularly relevant for creating motivating, challenging, playful and autonomous environments which are more likely to lead to long-term participation (Araújo et al., 2010; Côté et al., 2007; Renshaw et al., 2012; Côté, Erickson & Abernethy, 2013). Jumpers for goalposts and its concomitant iterations such as cage football are good examples of exploratory practice and sport experiences and deliberate play. The unstructured, emergent, and often self-regulated, notion of football is one that is appealing to many in a UK context.

3.4 Mass Games and Park Football (Us versus You)

A historical version of jumpers for goalposts is the mass, spontaneous games seen in parks up and down the country. For the football mad authors in this book brought up in the United Kingdom, as young players, we would often go for a 'pick up' game in the park, organising games against other boys (or girls) who were there, and this meant games were often against younger and older players. Often, when playing with younger players, we would invariably stack the odds against the older players by creating teams of uneven numbers. The idea was to get a balanced game or one where the better players had to work hard to win. If player numbers were low, rules would be adapted. For example, 'rush' goalies were introduced where the goalkeeper was not one fixed person and the nearest player to the goal would be allowed to use his/her hands. Uneven team numbers offer opportunities for variable technical and tactical solutions to emerge. For example, a team with lower numbers may solve the problem by developing their dribbling skills to cope with being confronted by two or more defenders. In contrast, the team with more players would be invited to exploit their numerical superiority by moving the ball quickly by developing a fast passing game and opportunity to counter quickly (especially if the other team had rush goalies and the goal was empty for a brief time). These games highlight how young players can learn to pick-up and exploit dynamic affordances that vary from game to game. An essential skill for these pick-up 'mass' game participants was the capacity to continually adapt rules with the goal of 'evening out' the game, which would often last for hours at a time. This extended 'practice time' provided multiple opportunities to develop technical, tactical (in the context of small-side games), physical and psycho-social skills (now the four corners of the English Football Association's 'DNA', see for example http://www.thefa.com/learning/coaching/the-fas-4-corner-model). These games would offer a wide landscape of affordances to be explored, with several layers of complexity present-ing numerous individual and co-adaptive interaction (between players) opportunities to promote players problem-solving ability in attempts to achieve the outcome goal which generally was about scoring more goals and often in a spectacular way. Here, players are implicitly embracing the ideas of repetition without repetition with the same goal in every ball possession, but the need to find new solutions each time, especially as opponents are often the same and they become attuned to the strengths and weaknesses of each other. Rather than this being a negative factor, this familiarity encourages exploration and cre-ativity and acts to increase the degeneracy of players. The result of these variable play opportunities is that perceptual, cognitive and physical processes are deeply intertwined as players are engaged in solving problems that arise from the emerging and decaying con-straints in a mass game. This is a really well-considered activity which has a strong basis in principles of Ecological Dynamics. The varying iterations of 'jumpers for goalposts' offer an interesting insight into the deliberate play, and developmental journeys of footballers in the United Kingdom.

In many parts of the United Kingdom, the notion of 'jumpers for goalposts' has all but disappeared but the philosophy and mentality remain valid. Andy Roxburgh (pre-viously the technical director for UEFA, https://web.archive.org/web/20170315001853/http://www.illinoisyouthsoccer.org/docs/CoachesHome/CoachesCorner/STREET%20SOCCER.pdf) wrote that 'The street game was player-centred, competitive, skilful and fair', providing an unstructured opportunity to play. A group of girls or boys putting down jumpers to act as goalposts, ascertaining the approximate height of the cross bar and agreeing what was in or out of the goal, was the cornerstone of talent development in UK football and helped to develop the skilful, physically fit, moral and strategic player. Similar to the young street basketballers of New York, youngsters in the United Kingdom often practice for hours using, developing tricks and skills, practicing with a friend or on their own endlessly reimagining a real game with nothing other than a ball, the wall or a pavement edge as a practice partner. In the next section we will discuss how street football shaped the skills of many great footballers by specifically focusing on a player coming towards the end of his career (Wayne Rooney) and one renowned as one of the greatest entertainers and still playing in the Premier league today (Wilf Zaha).

3.5 The Last of the Street Footballers?

Wayne Rooney amassed some 53 goals in 120 appearances for England and 253 goals in 559 appearances for Manchester United. Record scorer for both his country and one of the biggest clubs in world football. And whilst he was a product of an academy system, it is arguably not just that academy system but the streets of Croxteth where he grew up. His manager at Everton (his first club), David Moyes, once stated that 'he could play in goal, he could play as right back, he could play as a centre half, he could play as a midfielder. It was always because he was a footballer first. He was a genuine old-fashioned street footballer. I used to say, there wasn't many left' (Press Association – May 12, 2018 (https://www.thenational.ae/sport/football/last-of-the-street-footballers-david-moyes-pays-tribute-to-wayne-rooney-1.729589). Jason Burt, Telegraph columnist described Rooney as 'the last of the classic street footballers' and cites Rooney as stating that 'I've always believed myself to be from the streets in terms of football, I've always played on the streets with friends and still do now and again when I get time. I go and do that. That is where I learnt to play football. There was a lot of help along the way from the academy at Everton, but the majority of my football was learnt on the streets'. (https://www.telegraph.co.uk/sport/football/teams/england/11156017/Wayne-Rooney-reveals-that-he-likes-to-play-street-football-when-he-returns-home-to-Liverpool.html)

3.6 Cage Football and the Case of Wilf Zaha

A Guardian article in the United Kingdom suggested in 2016 that some 14% of all premier league players hail from a 10-mile radius in South London, where street football and the modern version of jumpers for goalposts, 'cage football' is a particular hotbed of talent (https://www.theguardian.com/football/blog/2016/jan/08/croydon-south-london-football-hot-bed-english-talent-crystal-palace). It is clear that the emergence of formalised projects such as the Elite Player Performance Plan (EPPP) has brought some structure and enhanced coaching numbers and quality, yet there is still a cry for a less sanitised and less audited notion of football, one where players are returning to the spirit of street football. This is being replicated in academies such as Manchester City, where there is an area for play and the development of physical literacy, or Ajax in Holland who have an Athletics Skill Model 'skills playground' to support the development of adaptability in motor skills. See example of a skill playground in Figure 3.2. Chris Wenker suggested that this playground supports the development of deliberate play due to the importance for supporting player development (https://trainingground.guru/articles/az-alkmaar-build-performance-playground). It is clear that as opportunities to play decline, and the professionalisation of coaching

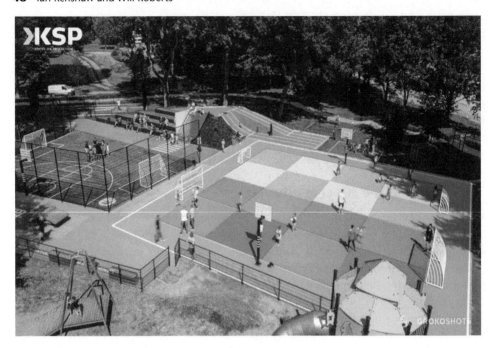

FIGURE 3.2 Cage football is the modern-day version of 'jumpers for goalposts' and is emerging as a hotbed for talented, creative footballers Street football in the United Kingdom. The photo is an example of ASM skills park.

increases, there are some challenges that we must address in order to expose young people to these opportunities to explore and hone skill in unstructured environments.

3.7 Pick-up Soccer in Brazil (Pelada)

Known as the 'People's Game', football (or soccer) is one of the most popular games played across continents. The FIFA World Cup is a huge spectacle that comes around every 4 years and footballing nations regardless of the level of football traditions aim to win the biggest prize (and honour). One nation, Brazil, with a proud record of winning the competition (5 times winner), has always captured the imagination of football fans around the world with their style and constant flow of world-class players in the Brazilian teams over the last 50 to 60 years. What is it in the culture of Brazilian football that provides such a constant pipeline of world-class players and teams? The answer could be found in how the game is played by millions of Brazilians in the streets of Sao Paolo, Rio De Janeiro or Belo Horizonte. The street version that is known as 'Pelada'.

Street games have a role in supporting elite athletes acquire the relevant skills and game play behaviours (Chow et al., 2015) and has always been intriguing for sports scientists in terms of its exact role in building expertise. Street games offer learning opportunities in natural settings and it is especially relevant in how these games offer players to exploit affordances in the natural and built environment. With reference to street football, it has been perceived as the most natural and spontaneous way of learning football (Garganta, 2006; Michels 2001; Scaglia, 2011, 2014; Garganta et al., 2013). Pelada is the kind of pick-up football termed in Brazil that are played in the cities and countryside and is very much a part of Brazilian culture (Uehara et al., 2018). In the cities, with tight space constraints, many of these games are played in hard concrete courts that are boxed up by metal fences (imagine a metal cage) called 'Quadras' (Borden, 2013, p. 11). Famous Brazilian legends of the game like Zico and Sócrates grew up with the unstructured but valuable learning environment provided by Pelada (Fonseca & Garganta, 2006, p. 12). These games are typically played in a space-constrained environment where 5 v 5 games are the norm. The speed of the game is fast and players are constantly challenged to move the ball quickly. Good close ball control is the order of the day and the ability to use the limited space afforded would be an advantage that any player could do with. There is obviously significant amount of time spent on the ball for players involved in these games and touches on the ball would clearly be significantly greater than in a typical 11-a-side game. One can also imagine the shooting opportunities afforded in these games. Teams flock to such 'quadras' to play the games and it is not uncommon for teams to wait for extended periods before getting involved in a game. Games could be played for a certain fixed period of time or when a team scores 3 goals first (Borden, 2013). It is case of survival of the fittest on many occasions and helps to create a high level of resilience and a winning mentality (if you want to stay in the game!). The level of competitiveness is intense and professional football club scouts are known to frequently watch some of these games in the hope of unearthing the next Ronaldinho or Neymar.

The characteristics of Pelada offers specific opportunities to develop players with a focus on skill with high temporal and spatial challenges that are representative of top-level football games. Machado et al. (2019, p. 13) captured some of the discussions on the advantage of being involved in such pick-up games in the form of Pelada (e.g., early familiarisation with ball, opportunities to exploit and explore varied movement solutions and high level

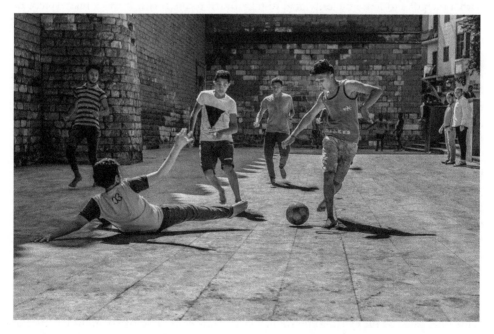

FIGURE 3.3   On the streets of Brazil, Pelada promotes dribbling, speed of thinking, flair and creativity that is a hallmark of Brazilian football

of autonomy are some of the stand out features offered by Pelada). A key benefit of playing these street games is that they provide players with copious opportunities to pick up surrounding perceptual information that affords different movement opportunities for different individuals (based on different intrinsic movement capabilities for the individual at that point in time) (Machado et al., 2019). The atmosphere of seeking to tease opponents by outrageous skill performance acts as an engine for skill adaptations and innovation (Uehara et al., 2018). The representativeness in the games is meaningful and individuals playing these games are presented with relevant perceptual information that constantly challenges them to search and exploit different ways to pass, dribble and shoot. Indeed, the time and space available in these games is very similar to that found in professional 11 v 11 football, and associated functional perception-action skills, when players take part in 'organised' football (Chow, 2013). The presence of teammates and opponents in tight space constraints also heightens the immense variability in actual game dynamics (task constraints) that cannot be replicated in more formal drill-based activities. These games promote dribbling, speed of thinking, flair and sometimes unpredictable movement adjustments that is a hallmark of Brazilian football (i.e., playing with the 'ginga' or sway and 'malandragem' or cunning and trickery) (Uehara et al., 2018). There are even suggestions that the *ginga* came about because of underlying racism where dark-skinned Brazilians were apprehensive about getting into physical contact with white players (and risk breaking a societal code) and thus the need to move their bodies in creative ways to actually glide around their white opponents with the ball! (Borden, 2013). Undoubtedly, Pelada games enable players to become attuned to and sensitive to key sources of information available in the game context (Renshaw et al., 2009, 2010, p. 15; Pinder et al., 2011, p. 14; Uehara et al., 2018). Take the example of how Ronaldo Luís Nazário de Lima, in the 2002 FIFA World Cup semi-final match against Turkey, weaved past a group of Turkish defenders and improvised with a toe poke to score the only goal to take Brazil to the finals. It was a masterpiece of spontaneous adjustment that could only be possible under that particular scenario where the perceptual information afforded him a toe poke as an emergent movement solution to achieve a successful outcome. The toe poke is uncommon in the context of the typical game as it may not necessarily provide the type of control in passing (or shooting) that is desired by players. But it is a functional movement skill in futsal. Enriched by previous experiences in futsal, at that moment, Ronaldo took what was possibly the only option available to him. Toe pokes do not allow the goalkeeper to anticipate an emerging shot from perceiving backswing information from the shooting limb in footballers. As well as futsal, the games of la pelada present such affordances on numerous occasions and the toe-poke is more common under the specific constraints of these street games than the 11-a-side game that typically offers more space and time for players to set themselves up for a pass or shot. Underlining the importance of physical literacy for athletic enrichment, the practice of many games, in different contexts, provides the players the opportunities to explore different game situations that are inherently unpredictable and variable. These experiences will encourage the players to co-adapt their performance behaviours according to emerging game constraints (Machado et al., 2019).

In a typical Pelada game setting, there are no coaches to formally direct and organise the players' activities. There is an absence of feedback given by anyone else. Participants adapt the game rules based on the existing environmental and task constraints based on the presence of obstacles (walls, gates, lampposts, bins) and different surfaces (ledges, pavements and kerbs). There are major opportunities for participants to express their autonomy and (for many young players) to perceive and solve problems that emerge in the game contexts (Machado et al., 2019). Self-directed learning becomes a necessity rather than an option. Players make 'mistakes' in these games but get to learn valuable lessons from those experiences that will help strengthen the critical perception-action couplings to promote more effectives action solutions in the longer term as can be seen from Figure 3.3. One cannot un-link the critical learner-environment mutuality that exists in all skill acquisition contexts (Renshaw & Chow, 2019). Importantly, the environmental constraints present in la pelada has been instrumental in producing such wonderful Brazilian players who have graced the world stage of football and have brought immense viewing joy for football fans around the globe.

3.8 Street Basketball in New York

Whilst football is the national sport in Brazil, in the five boroughs of New York (NY), basketball is the royalty of sports. According to its supporters, Street basketball is **the** NY urban game (Garica & Couliau, 2012). Whilst basketball was originally designed to be an indoor team sport, New Yorkers began to play the game outdoors on the streets and developed a style of play more in tune with the culture of the streets than the more passing-based game prevalent in organised competitions; the game changed from the 'pick and roll'

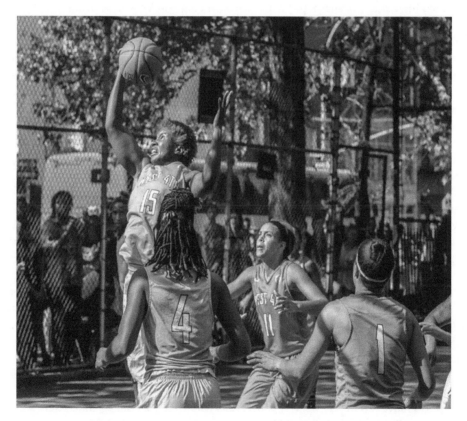

FIGURE 3.4   In the parks of New York, the interaction of culture, unique rules and game forms underpinning street basketball has led to the signature skills of New York basketballers, namely great ball handlers and outstanding shooters

and 'give and go' culture of professional basketball to a 'make it happen … the best way you can'. (Garcia and Couliau). As in Brazil, street culture influenced the way that the game was played, and according to Garica and Couliau individuals expressed themselves by bringing a 'street attitude' to the game. Street basketball became known as the City Game and the basketball equivalent of la pelada and became the breeding ground for future stars of the National Basketball Association (NBA). Whilst there were similarities in the games played in them, the culture and specific rules of each park were unique and consequently, players who moved across the boroughs in search of games or in a deliberate attempt to develop a city-wide reputation would have to adapt their game to the unique affordances of each playground. Thus, players had to become quick learners (see Chapter 1) and developed physical and mental skills that stood them in good stead in their later sporting careers.

In many of the more underprivileged areas of NY, the park is the communities' central meeting place and the way the game was played reflected the culture of mainly young African Americans. When communities 'live' outdoors, easy access to play areas can have a significant impact on the development of physical literacy as shown in Figure 3.4. Access provides an enriched and enabling environment for children and adults to acquire, adapt and maintain the requisite skills and capacities needed to sustain continued lifelong participation (Yeh et al., 2016) and enjoy the psycho-social and physiological benefits of participation. For example, in the Bronx in the 1970s, street basketball was played alongside the emerging culture of hip hop. Whilst breakdancing was viewed as being the physical expression of hip hop and graffiti art, the visual expression, basketball has also been viewed as the fifth element alongside DJing, MCing/rapping, breakdancing and graffiti (https:// www.youtube.com/watch?v=KCOm9LtYnaU). Basketball and hip hop had a symbiotic existence and influenced the way young disenfranchised Black African Americans dressed and acted around each other. It gave them the chance to express themselves and make a statement. It was, therefore, loud, brash and in-your-face. Hip-hop and basketball were both highly competitive and about one-upmanship. Gang culture was also influential and consequently, the way of life of street basketballers mirrored many of the characteristics of life on the street. Street basketball was all about demonstrating 'street attitude' and trash talking and embarrassing your opponent was just as important as winning. Former professional player and street ball legend of the 1960s James (Fly) Williams captured this neatly when he said: 'I gave no one no respect and I wasn't afraid of no one.' (https:// www.youtube.com/watch?v=Tu6yZboxPZo). Interviewed in Garcia and Couliau (2012) he further added: 'you had to live up to what you said' and 'pride was key, who you was (sic) and who you wanted to become'. Just like on the streets that surrounded the courts, hypermasculinity was paramount, and everything has to be earned and nothing was given. Only the toughest survive. Street basketball isn't laughing and joking, if there is laughing and joking it is not real basketball. As made clear by Richard (Pee Wee) Kirkland in Garcia and Couliau's documentary: 'you had to talk, go hard or go home, no zone [defence] was allowed" and 'it was man-to-man and you had to 'man-up". Just like in la pelada, there are no referees in street basketball and the game was highly physical, so you had to learn to play hard. Laughing and joking has no place in street 'ball and you learned to win 'by all means necessary'. Showmanship was a central part of the game and adding flavour to a move was highly valued by spectators who were watching games. Street legend Kenny and All American, 2 times NBA Champion (the Jet) Smith, emphasises this point, highlighting that: 'you are playing for the people on the side … it's all about the crowd" [which might be just one person]. Street basketball, therefore, became a focal point for the community and provided cheap entertainment. Flair and innovative play were rewarded with the socio-cultural constraints of 'performing' for others encouraging imaginative, problem-solving interactions to discover and exploit the surrounding information in the constantly changing dynamic pick-up game environments (see Chapter 1).

In the summer of 2012, Garcia and Couliau spent 90 days filming, listening and playing 'pick-up basketball' in the 180 courts in the five boroughs of New York. The film-makers describe pick-up basketball as 'happening when someone from a squad selects teammates from those who are there before the game starts'. As such, the game can be 1 v 1, 2 v 2, 3 v 3 or 5 v 5. These games are not governed by codified rules, there is no published start times and no schedules, no coaches or referees. The rules are unique to each local park and are not formally codified, written down or published online. According to Garcia and Couliau, a game begins when even a single player picks up a ball and starts to play and as such pick-up 'ball has no boundaries and it does not even need to be played on a court'. Games can be played on sidewalks, in alleys or against the walls of buildings. There is not even a need for 'proper' hoops with innovative youngsters using a coat hanger wire, a broken bicycle ring, monkey bars in the park, milk crates tied to a wall or even a dustbin as a basket. For those, who loved basketball, the court became their homes and players learned to adapt their games to heat and rain with games going on all day.

3.9 The Games

The games that players created depended on how many players were available for a game. If no one else was around, individual players developed speciality games to entertain themselves or use the opportunity to upskill themselves. These examples illustrate the culture of continuous enrichment and adaptation in a highly competitive, dynamic performance environment, which is an important tenet of physical literacy. For example, Geoff Huston, former guard for the New York Knicks, reporting playing his left hand against his right on a full court, up and down until someone else arrived. Players would give their games a name, for example, Ed Davis (AKA the 'Sundance Kid') who became a legend of the King Towers court in Harlem developed a game called 'The Sundance 15' where you had to shoot from 15 spots around the basket, meaning you had to practice shooting from all angles and distances. This game could be played alone or against others, often for money! One of the most popular games was 5-2, which developed into 21. Initially, 5-2 was a 1 v 1 game where one player would shoot from the edge of the key and a score was rewarded with 5 points and the opportunity to add another 2 points by scoring with the rebound. The player continued to shoot until he/she missed at which point his/her opponent got to shoot. The winner was the first player to make 52 points. Eventually, around the 1960s, defenders were added to the game which became known as 21, where it was one player versus 'the world', that is one player versus the rest of the players on the court. The winner was the first player to reach 21 points. The essence of the game was that you had to get through or get around the defenders and it meant that you had to develop your ball handling, your speed and quickness of thought. 21 made you a great ball handler and a shooter, which is what New York basketballers became known for in the parks and ultimately in the professional game. A key underpinning rule that ensured that pick-up basketball prepared players for the progression to professional basketball was the concept of 'next on'. In 5 v 5 pick-up basketball, the winning team (i.e., the first team to get to a specific score, e.g., 21) get to stay on court and play the next team which is made up from the people waiting. The structural mechanics of who goes on court is determined by who's got next. We discuss this rule and the implication for talent development in the following section.

3.10 Who's Got Next: A Meritocracy

Unlike other areas of life in New York, where you came from didn't matter with unconscious bias and discrimination having no influence on an individual's opportunity to succeed. On the playgrounds, who got to play was determined purely by ability. Consequently, pick-up basketball is all about inclusion and everyone is welcome to play, irrespective of age, gender, salary, colour, creed or religion. As reported in Garcia and Couliau's (2012) documentary, if you are good people and you come, you get the chance to play. However, to get on court, there is one requirement; you have to be good enough and every player has to 'earn the right' to play by demonstrating that he or she is good enough. A good example to illustrate this point, was Kenny (The Jet) Smith who ultimately became an All American and 2 times NBA Champion. Smith reflects that he didn't get on the main court in his own locale until he was 15, as he wasn't good enough. Consequently, to get on court, Smith reported spending hours and hours practicing …'all day, trash talking yourself, no refs, [learning] to hold your own [despite] … illegal methods, physical and verbal assaults to try and intimidate you' (Garcia and Couliau). Simply getting on court and then actually winning was, therefore, seen as a major milestone and a significant achievement as highlighted by Smith, stating that the first time he won on the main court in his own area[DK19] was the greatest memory in his whole basketball career. So, why is it so difficult to get on court? Surely, the next five players who had been waiting for the longest time would simply be next on once a game finished? Well in New York, street basketball, this was not the case and who got to go on court was determined by whoever had 'next'. Whilst, generally this was the player who has been waiting the longest, there was one proviso; if you had 'no game', you never called next as you wouldn't want to get on the court to be smashed. You also had to be known or other players would take 'next' off you. So, presuming a player was good enough and got to call 'next', what does the privilege mean? Essentially, he or she gets to pick the other four players to go on the court and he or she would only select players who would fight for the court with the goal of staying on for as long as possible. At popular times, courts can have up to 50 players waiting for a game, so if you aren't next, you need to be known *and* in the best four out of that 50.

This requirement ensured that even to get on the court, a player has to continually develop and put the work in, especially needing to develop resilience. The importance of winning to carry on playing also meant learning to play hard and created a culture where toughness was required and expected. As reported in the documentary, if a player hadn't ever left the basketball crying and bleeding then he/she had not 'served their time'. Some players had ambitions to become 'street legends and to get a city wide 'rep' and to achieve this would travel around and hunt down competition. The goal was to dominate the parks by going to a playground, find out who the best player on a court was and take him on. Clearly, the culture of street basketball created a set of affordances that promoted the requirement for ambitious young players to undertake many hours of competition and practice). However, rather than deliberate practice (Ericsson, Krampe & Tesch-Römer, 1993), achieving success on the courts of NY required high levels of variable practice (i.e., 'repetition without repetition' and dexterity (Bernstein, 1967) to exploit high levels of degeneracy to exploit and satisfy a wide range of task and environmental constraints. On a psychological level, success also required significant levels of 'resilience' or 'perseverance' and self-regulation to invest in improvement. From our perspective, this route is more likely to produce champions than the early selection models currently being followed by many professional sporting organisations. It is also more likely that those seeking to find 'talent' would have much more success by accessing this 'talent pathway' as it is more likely to reveal those individuals who have the capacity to undertake the significant levels of commitment needed to reach high levels of expertise. Of course, the corollary to this shift in timing of talent selection is that talent identification and selection would be much more efficient and give children the time and space to develop their skills without the goal of 'making it' inherent in current structured talent pathway programmes. Indeed, success in these environments did not go unnoticed and attracted the attention of scouts and coaches of pro teams who came to watch and pick players who had built up reputations.

The evidence supports the view that street basketball provides a rich landscape of affordances that can be explored and exploited to prepare players for future success in professional basketball. Many famous NBA players began their careers playing street basketball and credit their success as being down to the tough grounding inherent in street basketball as being central to the mental and technical skills that got them to the top. These ideas are captured by former NBA great, Corrie (Homicide) Williams who highlighted in Garcia and Couliau (2012) that he 'learned everything that made him the player he became through street basketball, not university basketball'. He added 'I was so bad at 13, that even if I was only one of 10 players on the playground, I wouldn't get on court'.

It should be clear from the narrative in the previous section that socio-cultural constraints of locales have a significant impact on the emergence of functional co-adaptability through the interactions with unique landscapes of affordances. The task and environmental constraints of such surroundings provide an ideal landscape to continue the physical literacy journey of children and youth in specific contexts of street football and basketball. A consequence of these dynamic interacting constraints is the game(s) of choice of children. In New York, street basketball is *the* game and for many youngsters, their heroes are those who play in the parks, not NBA stars. Great street players attracted huge crowds and it was 'ShowTime'. Modelling effects were apparent as spectators left enthused with the desire to make it onto the court. Consequently, youngsters were attracted to the parks in the quest to emulate their heroes. Street ball also shapes player's games and enables holistic development that enhances all of their physical, psycho-social and emotional capacities that can underpin a lifelong engagement in physical activities such as basketball. Dr. James Naismith, the inventor of basketball, famously said that basketball was a game that could not be coached, [DK20] but could only be played (https://youreduchoices. blogspot.com/2018/06/james-naismith.html). Street basketball reflects these goals and for advocates is seen as the purest and most unsullied version of the game (Garcia & Couliau, 2012). Indeed, it could be argued that for many, street basketball is where their roots grew from and the popularity associated with modern-day professional basketball such as the NBA owes its success to street basketball. For those who love basketball, pick-up is the true game as it can be played for life, having the potential to enrich individuals' behaviours throughout the period from childhood to older adulthood. As highlighted by Garcia and Couliau (2012) those who play street basketball do it wholeheartedly and for the love … all day long! Clearly, street basketball meets the basic psychological needs of its participants and as Geoff Huston, says years after retiring from professional basketball; 'when I hear the ball bounce I get chills'… 'I love basketball'. 'I can do it all day long'.

3.11 Conclusion

In Chapter 1, we argued that the 'power of play' has the potential to transform children's lives by helping them to combat stressors of modern life and enhance their capacity for learning. This claim became more significant and indeed 'obvious' during the recent COVID-19 lockdown. Being locked down for most of the day, and the sheer numbers of all generations teeming into the parks on being 'let-out' at the end of the day highlighted that children (and parents) have an innate need to play and engage with our natural environments.

However, as predicted by Kaplan as long ago as 1991 and Whitehead in 1993, (see Chapter 1), children of the 2020s continue to have fewer and fewer opportunities to direct their own play through the combined effects of more stringent educational testing regimes at early ages, lack of opportunity to spend time outdoors in local parks and backyards as parents work longer and longer hours and additionally by our focus on organised sport for younger and younger children. Additionally, the emergence of smartphones and laptops and online video games exacerbates the problem as exemplified by the huge growth in e-sports, which invite children to stay indoors to 'compete' (although see Polman et al., 2018 who argue that the emergence of e-sports has the potential to influence health outcomes across the lifespan and address some of the major barriers to current physical activity patterns).

In this chapter we have argued that children are being denied the opportunity to develop the essential physical literacy skills that underpin lifelong enjoyment and engagement in sport and physical activity. However, we have demonstrated that potential solutions are available if we simply go 'back to the future' and deliberately design-in opportunities for children to play backyard games. To that end, we strongly believe that creating local and accessible play environments that invite children (and adults) to become embedded in landscapes of affordances that allow them to explore and innovate is an essential requirement in local communities. Designing-in such environments should become a priority for local authorities and could act to promote short, medium and long-term engagement in physical activity and sport for all, irrespective of age or ability. At the same time, we believe that the empiric evidence shows that unstructured play has the capability to provide the foundation stones for those pursuing excellence.

We began this chapter by highlighting the important place of play as the foundation for learning in sports but noted that opportunities to play have been reduced over time. We suggested that contributing factors could include the combined effect of lack of time due to the pace of life as parents are forced to work longer hours, fewer physical places to play, the earlier focus on academic work for children, as well as the emergence of computers as play partners. Additionally, children are submitted to more adult-directed learning activities which they (the adults) see as more 'useful' in helping children develop expertise than 'wasting time' simply playing. A final point we made is that the early specialisation strategy of capturing children at a young age, adopted by many sports organisations, is exacerbating the problem, as adults have introduced organised sport to teach youngsters how to play games and sports 'properly' at younger and younger ages. However, if the goal of these programmes is to produce more and 'better' players, then they are simply not working. We then discussed how playing games in 'natural' environments such as backyards, streets and parks children (and adults) with the affordances could support their long-term development towards potential expertise. For example, these informal games invite hour upon hour of engagement and participation, irrespective of unfavourable weather conditions. Winning is important in these environments and often the rules encourage players to work hard on their skills 'outside' of the games themselves. Basically, in la pelada and street basketball, to be picked you have to be good enough, so extra work on skills is essential if you want to get on court. Similarly, in other sports like backyard cricket (see Chapter 12), sibling or peer rivalries are often a key driver in creating fierce competition. Often, environments act to shape the signature skills of individuals and help create points of difference between them and their rivals later down the line. Freedom from adult control allows high levels of exploration and leads to adaptable performance via dexterous actions. Whilst la pelada, jumpers for goalposts and backyard cricket games are categorised as unstructured play, often these environments are shaped by unwritten rules that provide a significant level of structure that drives the way participants act in them.

So, given the benefits of learning in natural environments and the reduced amount of play being experienced by youngsters, is (in our experience of coach and teacher educators), impacting their ability to design games when they graduate to become teachers and coaches, what can we do to help 'bring back play'? Interestingly, when I (Renshaw) lead coach or teacher education courses and invite participants to discuss the role of backyard games by asking them to talk about their own learning, the room comes alive and coaches and teachers become extremely animated in telling their own stories. All agree that the best learning was in backyard games, but the question, 'how should we bring the backyard into our practice?' leads to deafening silence. Clearly, despite their own experiences, there is still a disconnect for many practitioners between the benefits of 'proper' teaching and coaching and simply playing to learn. Or perhaps they are simply short of ideas?

References

Araújo, D., Fonseca, C., Davids, K. W., Garganta, J., Volossovitch, A., Brandão, R. & Krebs, R. (2010). The role of ecological constraints on expertise development. *Talent Development & Excellence, 2*(2), 165–179.

Barker, R. G. (1965). Explorations in ecological psychology. *American psychologist, 20*(1), 1.

Bernstein, N. A. (1967). *The co-ordination and regulation of movements.* Oxford, NY: Pergamon Press.

Borden, S. (2013). Pickup Soccer in Brazil Has an Allure All Its Own. Retrieved from https://www.nytimes.com/2013/10/20/sports/soccer/pickup-soccer-in-brazil-has-an-allure-all-its-own.html

Calvin, M. (2017). *No hunger in paradise: The players. The Journey. The Dream.* London: Random House.

Cannane, S. (2011). *First tests: Great Australian cricketers and the backyards that made them.* Australia: HarperCollins.

Chow, J. Y. (2013). Nonlinear learning underpinning pedagogy: Evidence, challenges and implications. *Quest, 65*, 469–484. doi:10.1080/00336297.2013.807746.

Chow, J. Y., Davids, K., Button, C. & Renshaw, I. (2015). *Nonlinear pedagogy in skill acquisition: An introduction.* London: Routledge.

Côté, J., Baker, J. & Abernethy, B. (2007). Practice and play in the development of sport expertise. *Handbook of Sport Psychology, 3*, 184–202.

Côté, J., Erickson, K. & Abernethy, B. (2013). Play and practice during childhood. In J. Côté & R. Lidor (Eds.), Conditions of children's talent development in sport (pp. 9–20). Morgantown, WV: Fitness Information Technology.

Coutinho, P., Mesquita, I., Davids, K., Fonseca, A. M. & Côté, J. (2016). How structured and unstructured sport activities aid the development of expertise in volleyball players. *Psychology of Sport and Exercise, 25*, 51–59.

Ericsson, K. A., Krampe, R. T. & Tesch-Römer, C. (1993). The role of deliberate practice in the acquisition of expert performance. *Psychological Review, 100*, 363.

Fonseca, H. & Garganta, J. (2006). Futebol de rua: um beco com saída: do jogo espontâneo à prática deliberada. Lisboa: visão e contextos.

Garganta, J. (2006). Ideias e competências para "pilotar" o jogo de Futebol. In Go Tani, J. Bento & R. Peterson (Eds.), Pedagogia do desporto (pp. 313–326). Rio de Janeiro: Guanabara Koogan.

Garganta, J., Guilherme, J., Barreira, D., Brito, J. & Rebelo, A. (2013). Fundamentos e práticas para o ensino e treino do futebol. In Fernando Tavares (Ed.), Jogos desportivos coletivos. Ensinar a jogar (pp. 199–263). Porto: Editora FADEUP.

Gibson, J. J. (1979). *The ecological approach to visual perception.* Boston, MA: Houghton, Mifflin and Company.

Jansson, M. (2010). Attractive playgrounds: Some factors affecting user interest and visiting patterns. *Landscape Research, 35*(1), 63–81.

Jongeneel, D., Withagen, R. & Zaal, F. T. (2015). Do children create standardized playgrounds? A study on the gap-crossing affordances of jumping stones. *Journal of Environmental Psychology, 44*, 45–52.

Machado, J. C., Barreira, D., Galatti, L., Chow, J.Y., Garganta, J. & Scaglia, A. J. (2019). Enhancing learning in the context of Street football: A case for nonlinear pedagogy. *Physical Education and Sport Pedagogy, 24*(2), 176–189.

Martens, R. (1978). *Joy and sadness in children's sports.* Champaign, IL: Human Kinetics Publishers.

Michels, R. (2001). *Team building: The road to success.* Spring City, PA: Reedswain.

Nebelong, H. (2004). Nature's playground. *Green Places, 5*(4), 28–31.

Phillips, E., Davids, K., Renshaw, I. & Portus, M. (2010). Expert performance in sport and the dynamics of talent development. *Sports Medicine, 40*(4), 271–283.

Pinder, R. A., Davids, K., Renshaw, I. & Araújo, D. (2011). Representative learning design and functionality of research and practice in sport. *Journal of Sport and Exercise Psychology, 33*(1), 146–155.

Polman, R., Trotter, M., Poulus, D. & Borkoles, E. (2018). *eSport: Friend or foe?* Paper presented at the Joint International Conference on Serious Games.

Renshaw, I. & Chappell, G. (2010). A constraints-led approach to talent development in cricket. In L. Kidman & B. J. Lombardo (Eds.), *Athlete-centred coaching: Developing decision makers* (pp. 151–172). Christchurch: IPC Print Resources.

Renshaw, I. & Chow, J.Y. (2019). A constraint-led approach to sport and physical education pedagogy. *Physical Education and Sport Pedagogy, 24*, 103–116. doi:10.1080/17408989.2018.1552676.

Renshaw, I., Chow, J.Y., Davids, K. & Hammond, J. (2010). A constraints-led perspective to understanding skill acquisition and game play: A basis for integration of motor learning theory and physical education praxis? *Physical Education and Sport Pedagogy, 15*(2), 117–137.

Renshaw, I., Davids, K., Phillips, E. & Kerherve, H. (2011). Developing talent in athletes as complex neurobiological systems. In J. Baker, S. Cobley & J. Schorer (Eds.), *Talent identification and development in sport: International perspectives.* London: Routledge.

Renshaw, I., Davids, K. W., Shuttleworth, R. & Chow, J.Y. (2009). Insights from ecological psychology and dynamical systems theory can underpin a philosophy of coaching. *International Journal of Sport Psychology, 40*(4), 540–602.

Rietveld, E. & Kiverstein, J. (2014). A rich landscape of affordances. *Ecological Psychology, 26*(4), 325–352.

Rothwell, M., Davids, K. & Stone, J. (2018). Harnessing socio-cultural constraints on athlete development to create a form of life. *Journal of Expertise, 1*(1), 94–102.

Rothwell, M., Stone, J. & Davids, K. (2019). Exploring forms of life in player development pathways: The case of British rugby league. *Journal of Motor Learning and Development, 7*(2), 242–260.

Rudd, J. R., Barnett, L. M., Butson, M. L., Farrow, D., Berry, J. & Polman, R. C. (2015). Fundamental movement skills are more than run, throw and catch: The role of stability skills. *PloS One, 10*. doi:10.1371/journal.pone.0140224.

Scaglia, A. J. (2014). Pedagogia do futebol: Construindo um currículo de formação para iniciação ao futebol em escolinhas. In Nista-Picollo Vilma & Toledo Eliana (Eds.), Abordagens Pedagógicas do Esporte: modalidades convencionais e não convencionais (pp. 16–67). Campinas: Papirus.

Soberlak, P. & Cote, J. (2003). The developmental activities of elite ice hockey players. *Journal of Applied Sport Psychology, 15*(1), 41–49.

Solomon, S. G. (2005). *American playgrounds: Revitalizing community space.* New England: UPNE.

Uehara, L., Button, C., Araújo, D., Renshaw, I. & Davids, K. (2018). The role of informal, unstructured practice in developing football expertise: The case of Brazilian Pelada. *Journal of Expertise, 1*(3), 162–180.

Vaughan, J., Mallet, C. J. & Davids, K. (2019). Developing Creativity to Enhance Human Potential in Sport: A Wicked Transdisciplinary Challenge. *Sheffield Hallam University Research Archive*, 2090. Retrieved from https://www.frontiersin.org/articles/10.3389/fpsyg.2019.02090/full?utm_source= F-NTF&utm_medium=EMLX&utm_campaign=PRD_FEOPS_20170000_ARTICLE

Whitehead, M. (1993). Physical Literacy. Unpublished paper presented at IAPESGW Congress, Melbourne, Australia.

Withagen, R., Araújo, D. & De Poel, H. J. (2017). Inviting affordances and agency. *New Ideas in Psychology, 45*, 11–18.

Withagen, R., De Poel, H. J., Araújo, D. & Pepping, G. J. (2012). Affordances can invite behavior: Reconsidering the relationship between affordances and agency. *New Ideas in Psychology, 30*(2), 250–258.

Yeh, H. P., Stone, J. A., Churchill, S. M., Wheat, J. S., Brymer, E. & Davids, K. (2016). Physical, psychological and emotional benefits of green physical activity: An ecological dynamics perspective. *Sports Medicine, 46*, 947–953. doi:10.1007/s40279-015-0374-z.

SECTION II

Contemporary Approaches for Operationalising Physical Literacy

Section 2: Introduction

The value of unstructured play, that is play which is not formally organised and managed by a system or a leader, is accepted across the expertise continuum. Evidence from ethnographic and observation-based research has revealed its importance for participation and recreational entertainment for inhabitants of lower socio-economic areas globally (Uehara et al., 2018). It has also been documented as fundamental for the development of football skills at the highest level of performance (e.g., Uehara et al., 2020). Theoretically, these research outcomes are well aligned with an Ecological Dynamics rationale for motor learning suggesting that a rich diet of structured and unstructured play and activities can enrich skill levels, motivation and confidence in learners (Renshaw & Chow, 2019; Button et al., 2020; Chow et al., 2020). Indeed, the contributions of unstructured and structured play activities can enhance the physical literacy of participants (children, athletes and recreationists) across the life course (Rudd et al., 2020; O'Sullivan et al., 2020). What then is the role of practitioners in physical education and sport? We believe that despite the need for a change in focus the role of practitioners in physical education and sports programmes has never been more important. But what we do need from them is an approach that offers a much more nuanced balance of intervention and design, rather than prescription (Chow et al., 2020). Utilising the Ecological Dynamics concept of physical literacy outlined in Chapter 2, the practitioner's role is to harness the principles of skill adaptation to the changing constraints that children experience outside of the sports hall, in their everyday lives, for example, when playing street games such as those exemplified in Chapter 3. The role of the practitioner is to enrich the learner's experience and enhance their physical literacy journey as espoused by Rudd et al. (2020). The Ecological Dynamics conceptualisation of physical literacy leads us to characterise it as a non-linear process where participants will participate in play, physical activities and movement experiences, if they are seen to be meaningful, and when they are encouraged to engage in exploration, search and adaptation. A key property of unstructured environments for play activities is that they provide opportunities (affordances) for 'safe uncertainty' in exploring challenging tasks (Renshaw & Chow, 2019; Chow et al., 2020). Learners feel safe in exploring these performance environments for solutions to the uncertainties encountered in these contexts. Next, we will turn to contemporary pedagogical models which can harness these environmental properties. These include a constraints-based approach to teaching and coaching (CLA), Nonlinear Pedagogy (NLP), Environmental Design Principles and the Athletic Skills Model.

These pedagogical frameworks suggest that successful learning designers and programme architects are those with the ability to design enriched playful environments that can foster physical literacy, they understand the importance of creating environments that lead participants on a journey of movement exploration and discovery and how this leads to learning in development. This is not to say that adult-led children's sport, physical education and physical activities that rely on heavily structured environments, are necessarily detrimental to learning *per se*, but as we will see in this chapter this is done under the assumption that our aim is to support children to master a particular movement skill through a process of automatisation. Contemporary theories of motor learning (Ecological Dynamics) inform us that this is not the case but instead results in high specificity of practice and may lead to learners becoming heavily dependent on teachers and coaches (practitioner) and a narrow focus, on the learning of a more specialised set of movement skills, which will result in the emergence of a limited field of stable coordination states (Chow et al., 2020). Whilst these coordination states will be stable and reliable in a specific performance context (e.g., during performance of a drill), this type of specificity will be rigid and inflexible and is less likely to support physical literacy, as it inhibits transfer across performance environments. Our goal in this section is to discuss how practitioners can be supported in operationalising physical literacy into their programme designs for children, youth sport and high-performance sport. This will mean practitioners need to ask some fundamental questions about their practice to support learn and acquire movement skills.

4

MOTOR LEARNING AND WHY IT MATTERS

How We Teach Physical Literacy

James Rudd and Keith Davids

4.1 Introduction

As we discussed in Chapter 2, Margaret Whitehead is responsible for the modern world-wide resurgence of interest in the concept of physical literacy. She has worked in, or around, physical education for the last 50 years and during this time came to believe that the subject of physical education had moved towards a high-level performance agenda and that this partly fuelled a perception in wider society that if you were not 'sporty' or involved in competitive sport then physical activity was not for you. David Kirk, echoed this concern, stating that pedagogy in physical education was not meaningful for the majority of children as more often than not physical education was being delivered as physical-education-as-sport technique, in other words, this is 'decontextualised physical education', that is, where practitioners deliver a multi-activity curriculum broken into short units in which pupils are introduced to isolated skills without the authentic sport/game experience and tactical aspects. In 2019, Kirk (2019) followed this up with an unflinching analysis that physical educators were unprepared to provide inclusive, fair and equitable forms of physical education that might empower young people to overcome the mal effects of precarity in today's society. He goes on to argue that now more than ever physical educators need to be 'alive' to the serious social and economic challenges that shape young people's health, happiness and life chances. Youth sport and high-performance coaching has not helped this image with its deliberate obsession with deliver practice (with not of) and the idea that it is 'essential' to undertake an average of 10,000 hours of intense practice that shouldn't be fun or involve games, but instead isolate skill development to focus on weaknesses (Ericsson, Krampe & Tesch-Römer, 1993). Our aim in this chapter is to provide a contemporary solution to this problem where the learner is placed at the core of the educational experience through the introduction of the Constraints-Led Approach (CLA) and to representative co-design. Before doing this, however, we will first revisit traditional approaches to motor learning and look at how these may have had an adverse effect on the direction of physical education and sport pedagogy through their advocacy for practitioner centred and directed approaches to physical education and youth sport teaching. Finally, we will offer an example of how adopting an Ecological Dynamics conceptualisation to physical literacy can ensure that we are better attuned the needs of children in today's society.

4.2 Motor Learning in the Last Decades and How It Has Shaped and Influenced Pedagogical Delivery

For much of the 20th century, the dominant theories of skill learning were stage theories of learning and information processing theory. Information processing theory suggests that information enters through the sensory system (e.g., visual, auditory, proprioceptive) and, similar to the way a computer works, it is encoded and stored in either our short- or long-term memory, depending upon the importance of the information. The central nervous system acts as the 'hardware' whose function is to order, monitor, select and organise the information, which dictates an internalised prescription of movement, coded as symbolic knowledge structures. Information processing theory postulates a top-down approach to movement with a construct located inside the brain, such as a schema or a mental representation, which is built up, or strengthened, as a result of the learning process so that a plan of action can occur before a movement emerges. This approach holds with the premise that learning is reflective of the maturation of a mental model and is a gradual linear process. Children become skilled movers through repetition of a skill, whilst development of a skill progresses through three observable stages of learning. In early learning the learner is thought to be in the cognitive stage of learning, where one learns about the movement execution through verbal instructions from a parent or practitioner, performing only some parts of a movement, which costs a lot of attentional effort. In the next phase, believed to be the associative phase, there is more refinement and improved control, which needs less conscious control, whilst movement execution requires less effort. In the third and final phase, automaticity of movement control is putatively achieved, providing room to perform other tasks in addition to, and at the same time as, the main movement this phase is aptly called the automatic phase. This traditional approach to the motor learning process has led to the belief that to teach movement skills requires a qualified supervisor, teacher or coach to prescribe a putative 'ideal' movement pattern and reduce any deviations from these technical templates. This model of learning is still dominant in the daily practical teaching of motor skills in physical education and sports programmes today. The lead author of this book regularly attends school physical education and youth sport sessions and more often than not the lessons follow an all too familiar format. They are overly structured by being divided into the format of an introductory activity, followed by a skill/drill practice phase focused on repetition of rote skills for developing and improving technique or aspects of technique. When the children have mastered the skill, they finish with a game or, as in the lesson plan in Figure 4.1, a gymnastics performance (Blomqvist, Luhtanen & Laakso, 2001).

The main aim of this performance pedagogy is to teach 'technical proficiency' (Oslin & Mitchell, 2006, p. 627), as it emphasises a skills first orientation where skills are learned 'before the introduction of rules and game play'. This form of teaching practice has been characterised by what Light and Kentel (Light et al., 2010) call a 'hard masculinised pedagogy', where the teacher is an authoritative expert passing on objectified knowledge, resulting in a power imbalance between the teacher and the child/learner. The most significant effect of this is that it leaves little to no room for children to adapt and explore their environments. The teaching and learning experience for the child includes both prescriptive actions (following technical demonstrations and instructions from the teacher) and repetitive actions to try to replicate the optimal technique where variability is reduced until a performer can execute a motor skill efficiently and reliably (Schmidt et al., 2018). Verbal feedback is often a one-way process with the teacher telling the child what they are

Year 1: 5-6-Year-Old Children		Aim of National Curriculum (United Kingdom): Master basic movements including running, jumping, throwing and catching, as well as developing balance, agility and co-ordination, and begin to apply these in a range of activities
Lesson's outcome		Children will be able to demonstrate **mastery** in a **log roll** and in **rocking back and forward** and will be able to use these skills in a **gymnastic performance**
Activity	Time	Activity Description
Warm up	5min	Activity that aims to raise children's body temperature and links to skills mastered last week. Run around the hall when teacher calls out a balance, children will perform balance (learnt in previous week)
Activity 1: Log Roll	10min	1. The coach explains and demonstrates the starting position of the log roll: laying down on a mat with legs straight while keeping arms straight above the head. Each child practices the starting position while the coach moves around the class giving corrective feedback. 2. When the coach is happy that a child can master the basic shape of the log roll, he/she invites the child to start practicing rolling across the mat.
Activity 2: The Rock (Teaching progression for the forward roll)	15min	1. The coach explains and demonstrates the starting position: sitting down on a mat maintaining the hold of the legs pulled in tight to the chest. Children practice getting in and out of the position. 2. The coach explains and demonstrates rocking backwards until the base the neck touches the mat and then rocking forward while keeping the body tight in the starting position. Children practice the skill until they demonstrate mastery. 3. Children practice with a partner trying to synchronise their rocking, so they stand up together.
Final Activity: The Performance	15min	The coach asks children to create a routine on the mat that must include the two rolls learnt during the lesson and a motor skill learnt in previous weeks. 1. Children create their own routine. 2. The coach divides the class in pairs and children combine their routine. 3. Each pair of children show the routine to the class.
Cool down	5min	The coach asks to walk around the hall and progressively slow down the walking pace until stopping and sitting down on a mat, then the coach invites children to copy the mobility exercises he/she performs. The coach asks questions about what children experienced and what they learnt during the lesson.

FIGURE 4.1 Traditional gymnastics lesson common practice in physical education and teacher training

doing incorrectly and proposing a different (and better) way of skill development (for further information see Box 4.1). From the learners' perspective the experience can be highly prescriptive as they receive constant instructions/corrective feedback for reproducing forms of movements or patterns of play (Chen et al., 2008; Davids et al., 2012). It is arguable that the rigidity and one-size-fits-all nature of this approach leaves little room for highly adaptive, emotionally engaged and motivated children and leads instead to passive learning.

BOX 4.1: FOUR COMMON PEDAGOGICAL PRINCIPLES OFTEN SEEN IN CHILDREN'S COACHING AND PHYSICAL EDUCATION LESSONS WHOSE ROOTS CAN BE TRACED TO INFORMATION PROCESSING THEORY

1. There is a correct optimal movement pattern for each movement skill.

   How it is linked to Information Processing theory: This is based on the idea that is there is a movement schema for each skill (blueprint) that acts as a reference of correctness to guide a child's movement.

   What we see in practice: The coach relies heavily on demonstrations of an optimal movement pattern as this offers an opportunity for learners to gather information about appropriate coordination patterns and task requirements which can benefit performance.

2. Movement skills are broken down or simplified into key components of a skill for learning, as performing an optimal movement pattern is often beyond the reach of children who are in the early stage of learning a skill.

   How it is linked to Information Processing theory: Linked to Fitts and Posner cognitive stage of learning, which costs a lot of attentional effort and so if we break down the skill into key components this requires less attentional (cognitive) effort.

   What we see in practice: Learning skill in closed environments free of environmental information. An example in football would be dribbling balls around cone before bringing in an active defender.

3. Movement variability (or error) is viewed as noise in the system, which the child has to reduce in their quest toward mastery of a skill.

   How it is linked to Information Processing theory: Again linked to Fitts and Posner's stages of learning where the end goal is for a skill to be automatic

   What we see in practice: The coach instructs repetitive practice of the skills, which gradually reduces the amount of variability in the system, the aim is an efficient, reliable and accurate movement skill performance.

4. Focus of attention when performing a movement skill can be implicit or explicit and is dependent on what stage of learning a child is currently in.

   How it is linked to Information Processing theory: Linked to Fitts and Posner model, during the cognitive phase of movement skill learning an internal focus of attention has been found to be advantageous reduces cognitive load. (see Beilock et al., 2002). Whilst in the associative and autonomous stage of learning an external attention of focus is advantageous (Wulf et al., 2013)

4.3 Contemporary Pedagogical Practice

As we have already noted, attention to contemporary theories of motor learning and development (e.g., Ecological Dynamics; Newell CLA, 1986; Smith & Thelen's work on dynamic system theory (Smith et al., 1995)) has, over the last 25 years, initiated a new focus on learning designs. These alternative forms of learning do not necessarily need the presence of a qualified supervisor but can be realised by creating environments that 'guide' and 'challenge' the child or athlete in such a way that desirable movement outcomes will be achieved. Underpinning the design of these environments is the aim to support learning as a process of discovering, exploring and improving motor skills. The practitioner's role is to design learning experiences in which the child's effectivities and capability and environmental opportunities are closely aligned. The child is left free to experiment by performing, adapting and creating the movement solutions that best answer their individual needs within a given context. The practitioner employs a range of different teaching techniques such as questioning the child. This not only opens up the teaching moment to allow for two-way communication but also encourages the child to problem solve and explore other functional movement patterns, promoting movement creativity.

4.4 The Constraints-Led Approach

The CLA is an important methodology that practitioners can use to help learners adapt their movements to the tasks and environments in which they are performing (Davids et al., 1994; Handford et al., 1997; Davids et al., 2008; Button et al., 2020). The CLA is based on Karl Newell's (1986) model of interacting constraints. He defined these as boundaries or characteristics that influence the coordinated state that emerges whilst a learner searches for a functional state of organisation, that is, a state of organisation that will allow each individual to achieve a specific task goal. Two important points to note from Newell's (1986) model of interacting constraints are: (i) the key implication that practice is a process of search for task solutions and (ii) the main goal of a learner in play, sport, physical education and movement more generally is to satisfy the immediate constraints acting on them. Satisfying impinging constraints is key to the 'functionality' of an individual. Functionality implies being able to make sense of a particular performance context and then to carry out relevant tasks and activities that an individual intends to complete. Constraints reduce the number of configurations available to a complex, dynamical system at any instance. They help to structure the number of possible system configurations for an individual. There are many classes of constraints that can shape the behaviours of a complex dynamical system, and it has been well documented that Newell (1986) considered personal (termed 'organismic'), task and environmental constraints to be the most influential (see Figure 4.2). Constraints refer to the characteristics of each

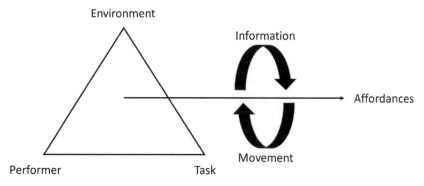

FIGURE 4.2 Newell's model of interacting constraints illustrates the cyclical process of perception and action

individual, such as genes, height, weight, muscle-fat ratio and cognitions and patterns of thinking, amount of previous experience and learning, motivation, emotions, feelings, desires. They need to be considered carefully by teachers and coaches since such personal constraints vary between, and within, each individual over different timescales. They can be influenced by factors operating over timescales of learning (hours, days, weeks) and maturation, ageing and development (months and years). Environment constraints are more global, and can consist of physical variables in nature, such as ambient light, temperature or altitude, or social features such as historical, cultural and societal values, beliefs and customs. Task constraints are more specific to performance contexts than environmental constraints and include task goals, specific rules associated with an activity, use of activity-related implements or tools and particular surfaces or objects involved in performance (Davids et al., 2008). A broad range of varied movement and play experiences, not only during childhood and youth but also into adulthood, can help an individual maintain and enhance physical literacy to support their skilled adaptation to the environment (Button et al., 2020; Chow et al., 2020).

Fundamentally, a CLA highlights the non-linear interactions between a performer (individual), task and environment (Handford et al., 1997; Davids et al., 2008). In the CLA, more skillful performance emerges through self-organisation under constraints as individuals become perceptually attuned to the key information sources which can regulate their actions in specific performance environments (when performing or learning) (Chow, 2013). A distinguishing feature of the CLA is that its practice design and delivery is informed by principles of a Nonlinear Pedagogy (NLP) that will be discussed in Chapter 5.

4.5 Importance of Co-design in Pedagogical Design to Support Physical Literacy

A central tenet of lesson, or session preparation, across the sporting landscape (from physical education to high-performance sports) is the appreciation of the child's/athlete's needs being placed at its core (Woods et al., 2020). This approach is in stark contrast to the more traditional models discussed earlier, which have tended to place the practitioner at the centre of the instructional process (Handford et al., 1997). An important concept in contemporary approaches of Ecological Dynamics is that the practitioner and child, or athlete, are envisioned as working in unison to co-design learning environments replete with critical information sources that solicit affordance realisation. This will support the development of self-regulating perceptions, cognitions, emotions and actions. Contemporary models, CLA, NLP and the Athletic Skills Model (ASM) conceptualise child/athletes, and/or at a higher scale of analysis class or sports teams, as complex adaptive systems (Glazier & Davids, 2009; Komar et al., 2015). In complex adaptive systems, learning results in synergy formation (i.e., coordination and adaptations) between system components, such as muscles, joints and limb segments and synaptic connections in the brain, or between members of a class or sports team, resulting in functional performance adaptations (Glazier & Davids, 2009). Synergy formation in complex adaptive systems is shaped bidirectionally: locally between the children or teammates themselves or externally, shaped by practitioners (Ribeiro et al., 2019). For practitioners observing children and athletes in a physical education lesson, or in performance preparation, it is important to understand how different types of constraints (related to the task, individual and environment) converge to facilitate synergy formation for realising novel affordances. In Ecological Dynamics, learning involves constraints-induced synergy formation between players, or parts of the body, through exploration, invention and adaptation of action possibilities (Glazier & Davids, 2009; Davids et al., 2012). Rich experiential knowledge from the child or athlete and practitioner can assist with the exploitation of bidirectional synergy formation (i.e., emphasising self-organising and self-regulating tendencies in athletes and teams, as well as the external influences of sport practitioners) (see Ribeiro et al., 2019). To exemplify, a practitioner may offer experiential knowledge that can guide the design of global 'principles of play' for children this could be simple safety rules to prevent accidents, whilst for athletes this might be to emphasise a full court press in basketball. Both of these show the way but are flexible to synergy formation from global to local-levels. In contrast, the child/athlete could provide a rich context to these principles based on their current action capabilities, what information is being detected, and insights into the most soliciting affordances they perceive to be available for use within the performance environment. This is likely to drive local self-regulating interactions and collaboration (between class/teammates) leading to the emergence of global behavioural patterns (Ribeiro et al., 2019). The presence of collaboration in the environment is crucial if we are to attend to a more holistic physical literacy journey for our learners. A learner's interactions with teammates and opponents within an environment will have the biggest impact on the self-organisation process. As learners attempt to achieve their task goal, they must collaborate with their teammates as they self-organise against the interacting constraints. This continuous process has been characterised as co-adaptation, with each learner's behaviours constrained by the information from the actions of the other learners in the environment (Passos, Araújo & Davids, 2016). Practitioners should avoid setting problems for learners to solve in environments devoid of other learners. Task constraints must be manipulated to provide learners with the opportunity to collaborate and co-adapt. It is important for the learners to develop an understanding of how their interaction with others within the environment can impact on both their own development, and upon others. Through the manipulation of task constraints, we can shift the emphasis from individual competition onto collaboration. This perspective uncovers an important feature of representative co-design in developing collaborative principles of play at high end performance sport where tactics perceived as important to overcome specific opponents, or performance challenges, are no longer considered to be the sole domain of the coach (Ribeiro et al., 2019).

Framed through representative co-design, intelligent athletes and coaches work together to share rich experiential knowledge surrounding performance principles or tactics. Indeed, such principles are developed with the players' needs and action capabilities placed at the core – fostering greater player engagement, self-regulation and ownership of the learning and preparation environment. Thus, instead of offering putatively 'optimised', 'ready-made' and pre-programmed task solutions (according to personal preferences), a coach would work with the athlete to develop individualised and creative solutions for performance problems, which are continually evolving in line with tactical developments in a sport. In this way, both coaches and athletes find solutions to the emergent problems encountered in dynamic competitive performance environments together (Araújo et al., 2009). The idea of representative co-design enjoins high-performance sport and physical education together, not with a focus on skill mastery or the masculine 'survival of fittest' mantra of performance sport that may have put previous generations off being physically active, but through enriching both ends of the performance landscape with the productive development of 'intelligent' performers. This should not be a big challenge for physical education as across the globe, government publications, national standards, professional bodies and curriculum documents in education have recognised that the development of intelligent performers needs to start in childhood, emphasising the role of problem-solving, thinking and decision-making skills in physical education. For example, the UK's National Curriculum Physical Education, the USA's NASPE (National Association for Sport and Physical Education) and the Queensland Physical Education Senior Syllabus (Queensland Studies Authority, 2010), incorporate this outcome in all three of the major domains of learning: psychomotor, cognitive and affective (see also National Association for Sport & Physical Education, 2009; Queensland Studies Authority, 2010; the Department for Education, 2013;). Notably, the Studies Authority in Queensland, Australia (2010, p. 3) states that: 'Intelligent performance is characterised by high levels of cognitive functioning, using both rational and creative thought. Students are decision-makers engaged in the active construction of meaning through processing information related to their personal experience and to the study of physical activity'. Existing ideas on intelligent performers across the sporting landscape are well aligned with connotations of physical literacy. The following three chapters provide pedagogical practices that can further bring all aspects of the sporting landscape closer together.

To conclude this chapter, we are keen to demonstrate how a deep understanding of Ecological Dynamics and placing a child's physical literacy journey at the heart of this can radically shift how we approach educating children in physical education. We believe that traditional approaches to physical education that contain smatterings of information processing theory are not fit for purpose in our current society. An educator who approaches a child's education through an Ecological Dynamics conceptualisation will first ask the question, 'does physical education educate children to their world?' This means that we need to recognise that children are situated in an ecological niche, that is their home environment, in which they have access to particular play spaces (garden, park or sports club) and that this is the landscape that they are currently (self)navigating to find their path shaping their ongoing physical literacy. The landscapes that we exploit or design in our physical education lessons must therefore help them with their wayfinding in the world that they inhabit. An example of this is teaching children to swim, which is a key aim of physical education curriculums across the globe. Based upon an Ecological Dynamics understanding of perception, action and affordances, learning to swim in the tepid/warm, calm water found at your local, brightly lit swimming baths may not actually address the need for all children to learn to swim. Across the globe children and adolescents make up the highest percentage of deaths by drowning and the vast majority of these events occur in open water, the sea, lakes, ponds and rivers.

Physical educators should therefore appreciate that whilst supporting children to perfect their swimming strokes like a Michael Phelps, or a Cate Campbell is a wonderful aspiration, this is for most children neither achievable, nor essential. A major take-home message from a physical literacy conceptualised Ecological Dynamics rationale is that technique reproduction should not be a major focus for children in the physical education setting, instead, we should understand that every child needs to have *knowledge of* different

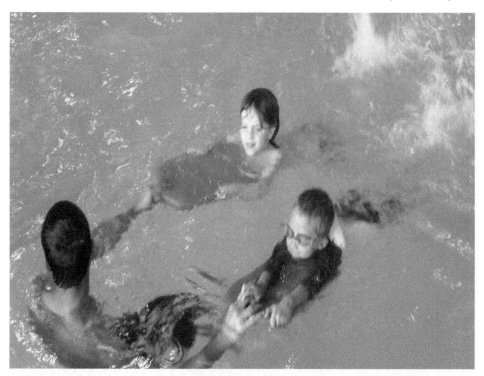

FIGURE 4.3   Two children being supported to swim using traditional methods. Task decomposed and it could even be argued that the girl is passively engaged in the learning process

aquatic (enclosed and open) water environments so he/she can self-regulate safely both around and immersed in such contexts. This is because educators who are learned in Ecological Dynamics understand that drowning is a multifaceted and complex phenomenon and is a consequence of the way a child interacts with their aquatic environment (Moran, 2007). Button, Schofield and Croft (2016) have demonstrated that children who learn survival skills in open water environments develop self-regulation tendencies, enriched by perceptual, cognitive, emotional and physical systems, leading to enhanced survival competencies and skills in only one or two lessons. Swimming pools are highly controlled environments, which mitigate risks as the pool's water temperature does not fluctuate, the surface remains in quasi-steady state and the downward slope is predictable (see Figure 4.3). The net result is that *knowledge of* the environment is minimal and does not transfer. This is in stark contrast to open water environments where currents, rips, waves, water depths and light levels and temperatures constantly fluctuate.

The environmental dynamics will (re)specify movements (e.g., the child to tread water, to estimate the duration between two waves, dive to avoid a crashing wave, or float to take benefit from the current or rip and experience different colours of depths) (see Figure 4.4). The *knowledge of* the environment gained in open water offers a rich landscape of affordances (e.g., waves, currents, rips, obstacles, low visibility) that invites learners to explore and to adapt continuously, which favour learner-environment coupling and is also transferable across these environments (Guignard et al., 2020). Transfer of learning is observed

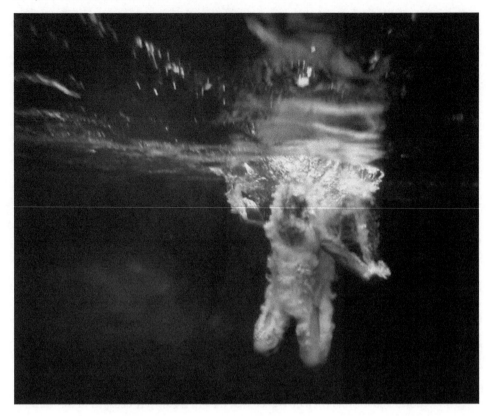

FIGURE 4.4 Contrast of open water environments where water temperature is very cold, dark and likely to contain unforeseen hazards

when children perform functionally in an untrained situation, as they are able to explore effectively and adapt their acquired skills to this new environment. Designing learning situations that are representative of the richness and complexity of open water environments goes beyond teaching swimming skills and should prioritise water safety skills (where at all possible taught in open water environments rather than in the pool), in order to guarantee that children can learn to transfer their skills across a variety of environments (Stallman et al. 2017; Guignard et al., 2020). In summary, water safety skills are enduring over time and, due to their relationship with available affordances in open water, they will be far more consequential in preventing death by drowning in children and adolescents compared to learning to swim in the tepid/warm, highly stable aquatic environment of a local indoor swimming pool.

4.6 Conclusion

The aims of this chapter were to begin to introduce a contemporary approach to physical education and sport that positions the learner at the core of the experience and to demonstrate how this supports physical literacy. We have investigated how in the past traditional theories of motor learning have shaped physical education and sports practices, putting the practitioner at the heart of the experience whilst children take on the role of passive learners on a journey to automaticity. We have seen that physical literacy is a journey of wayfinding that enables children and adults to develop a deeper knowledge of the environment, attaching value and meaning to activities through a process of exploration and adaptation. In this chapter we have begun to operationalise physical literacy through the introduction of contemporary pedagogical models derived from the concept of Ecological Dynamics. Specifically, we have introduced the CLA and the notion of representative co-design which we argue represent an important methodological advancement right across the sporting landscape from physical education to high-performance sport) by supporting a learner-centred approach that empowers performers, at all developmental stages, to take greater ownership of their learning.

References

Araujo, D., Davids, K.W., Chow, J.Y., Passos, P. & Raab, M. (2009). The development of decision making skill in sport: An ecological dynamics perspective. In *Perspectives on cognition and action in sport* (pp. 157–169). Nova Science Publishers, Inc., United States.

Blomqvist, M., Luhtanen, P. & Laakso, L. (2001). Comparison of two types of instruction in badminton. *European Journal of Physical Education, 6,* 139–155.

Button, C., Schofield, M. & Croft, J. (2016). Distance perception in an open water environment: Analysis of individual differences. *Attention, Perception, & Psychophysics, 78,* 915–922.

Button, C., Seifert, L., Chow, J.Y., Davids, K. & Araujo, D. (2020). *Dynamics of skill acquisition: An ecological dynamics approach.* Champaign, IL: Human Kinetics Publishers.

Chen, A., Martin, R., Ennis, C. D. & Sun, H. (2008). Content specificity of expectancy beliefs and task values in elementary physical education. *Research Quarterly for Exercise and Sport, 79,* 195–208.

Chow, J.-Y., Davids, K., Shuttleworth, R. & Araújo, D. (2020). Ecological dynamics and transfer from practice to performance in sport. In A. M. Williams & N. Hodges (Eds.), *Skill acquisition in sport: Research, theory and practice.* London: Routledge.

Davids, K., Araújo, D., Hristovski, R., Passos, P. & Chow, J.Y. (2012). Ecological dynamics and motor learning design in sport. In M. Williams & N. Hodges *(Eds.), Skill Acquisition in Sport: Research, Theory and Practice* (pp. 112–130). London: Routledge.

Davids, K. W., Button, C. & Bennett, S. J. (2008). *Dynamics of skill acquisition: A constraints-led approach.* Champaign, IL: Human Kinetics.

National Association for Sport and Physical Education. (2009). *National standards & guidelines for physical education teacher education.* National Association for Sport and Physical Education, Virginia, United States.

Ericsson, K. A., Krampe, R. T. & Tesch-Römer, C. (1993). The role of deliberate practice in the acquisition of expert performance. *Psychological Review, 100,* 363.

Glazier, P. S. & Davids, K. (2009). Constraints on the complete optimization of human motion. *Sports Medicine, 39,* 15–28.

Guignard, B., Button, C., Davids, K. & Seifert, L. (2020). Education and transfer of water competencies: An ecological dynamics approach. *European Physical Education Review, 26*(4), 1–16.

Handford, C., Davids, K., Bennett, S. & Button, C. (1997). Skill acquisition in sport: Some applications of an evolving practice ecology. *Journal of Sports Sciences, 15,* 621–640.

Kirk, D. (2019). *Precarity, critical pedagogy and physical education.* London: Routledge.

Komar, J., Chow, J.Y., Chollet, D. & Seifert, L. (2015). Neurobiological degeneracy: Supporting stability, flexibility and pluripotentiality in complex motor skill. *Acta Psychologica, 154,* 26–35.

Light, R., Kentel, J. A., Kehler, M. & Atkinson, M. (2010). Soft pedagogy for a hard sport: Disrupting hegemonic masculinity in high school rugby through feminist-informed pedagogy. In M. Kehlen & M. Atkinson (Eds.), *Boys' bodies: Speaking the unspoken* (pp. 133–154). Oxford, UK: Peter Lang Publishers.

Conceptualizing Physical Literacy within an Ecological Dynamics Framework. *Quest, 72*(4), 448-462. doi: 10.1080/00336297.2020.1799828.

Oslin, J. & Mitchell, S. (2006). Game-centred approaches to teaching physical education. In D. Kirk, D. Macdonald & M. O'Sullivan (Eds.), The handbook of physical education (pp. 627–651). London: Sage.

Passos, P., Araújo, D. & Davids, K. (2016). Competitiveness and the process of co-adaptation in team sport performance. *Frontiers in Psychology, 7*, 1562.

Queensland Studies Authority. (2010). Physical education senior syllabus. *Brisbane, Queensland, Australia: Queensland Studies Authority*.

Renshaw, I. & Chow, J.Y. (2019). A constraint-led approach to sport and physical education pedagogy. *Physical Education and Sport Pedagogy, 24*, 103–116.

Ribeiro, J. F., Davids, K., Araújo, D., Guilherme, J., Silva, P. & Garganta, J. (2019). Exploiting bi-directional self-organising tendencies in team sports: The role of the game model and tactical principles of play. *Frontiers in Psychology, 10*, 2213.

Rudd, J. R., Crotti, M., Fitton-Davies, K., O'Callaghan, L., Bardid, F., Utesch, T., Roberts, S., Boddy, L. M., Cronin, C. J. & Knowles, Z. (2020). Skill Acquisition Methods Fostering Physical Literacy in Early-Physical Education (SAMPLE-PE): Rationale and study protocol for a cluster randomized controlled trial in 5–6-year-old children from deprived areas of North West England. *Frontiers in Psychology, 11*, 1228.

Schmidt, R. A., Lee, T. D., Winstein, C., Wulf, G. & Zelaznik, H. N. (2018). *Motor control and learning: A behavioral emphasis*. Champaign, IL: Human kinetics.

Smith, L. B., McLin, D., Titzer, B. & Thelen, E. (1995). *The task dynamics of the A-not-B error*. Paper presented at the LB Smith (Chair), Tests of a dynamic systems theory: The object concept. Symposium conducted at the 1995 Meeting of the Society for Research in Child Development, Indianapolis, IN.

Stallman, R. K., Moran, K., Quan, L. & Langendorfer, S. (2017). From swimming skill to water competence: Towards a more inclusive drowning prevention future. *International Journal of Aquatic Research and Education, 10*, 3.

Uehara, L., Button, C., Araújo, D., Renshaw, I. & Davids, K. (2018). The role of informal, unstructured practice in developing football expertise: The case of Brazilian Pelada. *Journal of Expertise, 1*(3), 162–180.

Uehara, L., Button, C., Saunders, J., Araújo, D., Falcous, M. & Davids, K. (2020). Malandragem and Ginga: Socio-Cultural Constraints on the Development of Expertise and Skills in Brazilian Football. International Journal of Sport Science and Coaching. https://doi.org/10.1177/1747954120976271

WAID. (2018). Water Incident Database National Water Safety Report. Retrieved from https://www. nationalwatersafety.org.uk/waid/reports-and-data/

Woods, C. T., McKeown, I., Rothwell, M., Araújo, D., Robertson, S. & Davids, K. (2020). sport practitioners as sport ecology designers: How ecological dynamics has progressively changed perceptions of skill "Acquisition" in the sporting habitat. *Frontiers in Psychology, 11*. doi:10.3389%Fpsyg.2020.00654.

5

NONLINEAR PEDAGOGY

A New Framework for Designing Learning Environments for Sport, Physical Education and Recreational Activities

Jia Yi Chow

5.1 Introduction

Nonlinear Pedagogy (NLP) has been developed and constructed upon an Ecological Dynamics approach. At the heart of this pedagogical framework is exploratory learning, with an emphasis on encouraging individualised movement solutions. For this reason, it provides an excellent foundation for sport, physical education (PE) and recreational physical activity programme to support physical literacy. This is because accountability of learner-environmental mutuality is central to this approach. With reference to an Ecological Dynamics perspective, the processes of perception and action should be reframed as one that focuses on exploration and interaction. Teaching, coaching and learning must be underpinned by effective key pedagogical design principles that encourage learners to search for individualised movement solutions that are self-adjusted to satisfy the constraints present in the learning and performance environment (Chow, 2013). The focus is on the individual learner, and most importantly, how the learner interacts with the environment. The task itself is the platform where the learner and the environment continually interact to shape movement behaviours. 'Knowledge of the environment' rather that 'knowledge about the environment' becomes a key pillar for how physical literacy as reflected in Chapter 2 through wayfinding.

In this chapter, we will discuss the 'what', 'why' and 'how' of NLP and discuss how this framework relates to the enrichment of functional movement capacities which can underpin an individual's physical literacy, thus setting him/her up for a physically active lifestyle at specific performance levels from recreational to elite standards. Specifically, we address the following questions: (i) What is NLP? (ii) Why is NLP relevant? (iii) How can we apply NLP in practice contexts?

5.2 What Is Nonlinear Pedagogy?

Different individuals learn differently in different contexts. Even the same learner may display a myriad of behaviours in different learning environments. Undoubtedly, *nonlinearity in learning* can be observed across many skill acquisition/adaptation contexts. Typically, such nonlinearity in learning is common and not atypical. As pointed out in Chapter 2, children learn to perceive affordances at each moment, relative to their current intrinsic dynamics in the current performance environment and for the current task (Adolph & Hoch, 2019). The changes observed involves a non-linear process and the perception that children acquire functional movement skills at a steady rate is a fallacy. Chow et al. (2011) described some of the key features of nonlinearity and they relate to how: (i) we may observe non-proportionate changes (e.g., practising for a long time does not necessarily lead to an identical quantum of improvement: sometimes rapid jumps in learning can emerge from small periods of practice). In these instances, it is not reasonable to assume that the more a learner practices, the greater the amount of improvement there will be. Minor tweaks in the learning environment (e.g., different instructions or scaling of learning space and equipment) can lead to spontaneous jumps in performance and learning if the changes in task constraints can quickly direct the learner to discover new functional movement behaviours; (ii) there can be multiple ways to accomplish a task goal [e.g., one can kick a ball in different ways (instep, contact with the laces of the football boots or even a toe poke) as long as an intended outcome is achieved: e.g., the learner kicks the ball towards a target and scores a goal]. This relationship between performance process and outcomes has important implications for what expectations we should have of our learners in developing certain movement solutions to achieve a task goal and clearly has implications on how physical literacy is developed. It should signal the potential for learners to engage in an exploratory search (especially during play!) for different movement solutions; (iii) practitioners can scale task constraints and this approach can result in the emergence of new preferred movement behaviours (e.g., scaling the size of the ball can lead to different ways of catching it in a throw and catch game). Such scaling of task constraints can occur quite regularly in many teaching and coaching contexts and can inadvertently shape the emergence of different behaviours in a self-adjusted way and (iv) variability in practice can be an important factor in encouraging learners to move from one preferred movement behaviour to a new functional movement behaviour. It is through the presence of some quantum of variability in the learning environment that learners have the opportunity to adapt to this variation and try something different rather than attempting to repeat or rehearse a specific movement pattern in a drill. This clearly goes against the more traditional and previously accepted notion that repetitive drills to achieve a consistent single optimal movement pattern across different performance contexts is the gold standard (and perhaps the danger of early specialisation with an emphasis on repetitive drills!). Notably, variability in practice and in play is also typically observed under conditions where it would be almost impossible to repeat a movement in exactly the same way, for example, by regularly changing the positioning and type of hold on an indoor climbing wall.

5.3 What Is Meaningful Skill Adaptation?

Many observed behaviours that regularly emerge in various skill acquisition and adaptation contexts support the importance of accepting that features of nonlinearity in learning is inherent. Undoubtedly, if learners demonstrate such inherent tendencies, practitioners should consider pedagogical approaches that could account for such nonlinearity (Chow et al., 2016). The framework of NLP, with its design pedagogical principles and underpinned by the theoretical framework of Ecological Dynamics, can indeed be a viable approach to help practitioners make sense of how to engage learners and address the

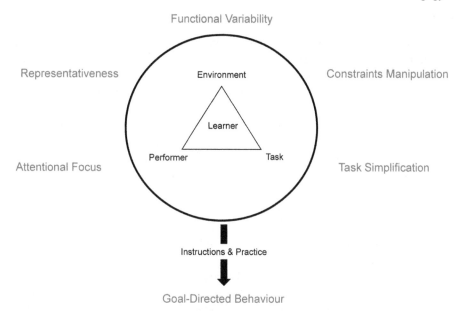

Functional Variability

Representativeness

Environment

Constraints Manipulation

Learner

Attentional Focus

Performer   Task

Task Simplification

Instructions & Practice

Goal-Directed Behaviour

FIGURE 5.1 Nonlinear Pedagogy approach featuring key pedagogical design principles

inherent nonlinearity in learning that is pervasive (Chow et al., in press). An understanding of the need for a pedagogical approach to account for nonlinearity in learning is critical for pedagogues and practitioners to consider appropriate design principles to support more effective learning. (Chow, 2013; Chow et al., 2016).

In NLP, the learner is at the centre of the NLP framework and importantly should be an active participant with autonomy to search and explore individualised movement solutions (Button et al., 2020; Chow, 2013). Learners should also be given opportunities to acquire individualised movement solutions based on the learning and performance context (Button et al., 2012; Hacques et al., 2020). See Figure 5.1.

Pedagogical design principles work through the channels of instructions and practice designs to support the emergence of movement behaviours (see Chow et al., 2013; Hacques et al., 2020; Ovens, Hopper & Butler, 2013). Research and theorising in NLP have demonstrated that the principles underlying NLP can be adopted to address the key question, 'What design principles can be used to support teaching and learning in Sports and PE?' (Chow, 2013; Correia et al., 2019). In this chapter, we discuss how practitioners can develop design principles that incorporate representativeness, manipulation of constraints, attentional focus, functional variability and the maintenance of pertinent information-movement couplings through task simplification (Chow, Davids, Renshaw, et al., 2020; Correia et al., 2019). These design principles support important discussion on how physical literacy is developed in learners as they are relevant in guiding practitioners in planning and enacting learning contexts where learner-environment mutuality is critical (Orth, van der Kamp & Button, 2019; Pinder & Renshaw, 2019; Roberts, Newcombe & Davids, 2019). It supports an embedded approach, which was highlighted in Chapter 2, to understanding skill acquisition and adaptation where task goals are achieved through interactions constrained by the body, task and environment (Renshaw & Chow, 2019).

5.4 Need for Representativeness in Practice

The inclusion of **Representative Learning Environments** for learners is based upon long-standing specificity of learning principles (see Henry, 1958). Importantly, specificity of learning necessitates representative learning designs (Button et al., 2020) and this is clearly relevant when the emphasis is on transfer of learning and meaningful skill adaptation, especially at higher expertise levels in sport. But what exactly does incorporating representative learning environments mean? It is certainly non-trivial and representative design requires a deep understanding of the information that constrains performance behaviours and the affordances that may invite specific functional actions needed by individual learners to achieve intended task goals (Chow, Davids, Renshaw, et al., 2020). The crux for ensuring representativeness in practice designs is to replicate and include relevant information and invitation for actions during the practice (Chow, Davids, Renshaw, et al., 2020). Specifically, learning activities should be situated in performance contexts that capture the dynamics where the skills to be learnt can be performed, developed and acquired. This may at first sight appear to be relatively easy to implement: why not just let the learners play the actual game or engage in the sport? Unfortunately, this approach is neither sensible nor feasible, especially when learning sports like mountain climbing or kayaking in white water. Deep thinking is required such that the practitioner must identify the key information sources and available affordances that can be amplified in representative learning activities to encourage learners to search and accept those invitations to act. The prevalence of symmetry designs in playgrounds, as described in Chapters 1 and 3, is a good example of the need to create representative learning environment. In the real world, it is unlikely that the environment would be structured with such high level of symmetry. Even the presumably simple act of walking across the road at pedestrian crossing points may offer challenges in the form of uneven road surfaces. Locomoting on asymmetrical platforms would indeed be more representative in learning contexts. Another example highlighted in Chapter 4 about learning to swim in a much-controlled environment in swimming pools versus open water challenges is relevant to the need to present representative learning activities. The water safety skills and swimming skills needed would be distinct for a learner exposed to learning environment in a swimming pool setting as compared to a lake or in the open sea. Closer to a sporting context, practising with and without opponents would also present different invitations to act. Perceptual information present in the environment would differ when a learner practices a serve in tennis without an opponent and may not be attuned to the value of serving to the part of the court that the opponent is not covering.

5.5 Constraints Manipulation

Practitioners should manipulate constraints (e.g., task constraints that include instructions, equipment and task goals) to encourage the demonstration of certain behaviours by the learners. The second key pedagogical principle relates to **Constraints Manipulation** and this basically underlies and supports many of the other design principles within NLP (Chow et al., in press). In the NLP framework, manipulating interacting constraints related to the learner, task and environment is a key consideration in understanding how goal-directed behaviours emerge.

For example, the scaling of key task constraints can support physical literacy of children by helping them to gain valuable experience in self-adjusting their emergent movement patterns (i.e., self-organisation of the learner-environment system in teaching and learning context) (Chow et al., in press). Task constraints can be intentionally manipulated or even scaled to channel learners to search and exploit different movement behaviours. However, the key here is intentional and purposeful manipulation of constraints (see Chow, 2013). For example, temporal and spatial constraints would be reduced with the use of a shorter racket and this could be easier for a novice picking up the sport of tennis (e.g., body-scaling to the anatomical constraints of a child). Similarly, a larger size ball would better afford catching with both hands, rather than one hand based on the interaction between the performer constraints (i.e., size of hand) and the task constraints (i.e., size of ball). Even the size of the grips of bar handles that we see at playgrounds would afford different play behaviours (e.g., smaller bar sizes or textured surfaces on the bar allows for easier grips as compared to larger ones or smoother handles).

Research has provided some evidence for the effectiveness of learning designs that manipulate key task constraints. This approach can be instrumental in enhancing an individual's physical literacy if they are well-considered to promote adaptive skill behaviours during search activities by learners. For example, a study conducted by Fitzpatrick, Davids and Stone (2017) in children's mini-tennis games, showed how manipulating key constraints in a thoughtful way could enrich the coordination of difficult actions like a backhand drive. Fitzpatrick et al. (2017) targeted key task constraints in children's tennis, including scoring format, court playing area dimensions, net height and ball characteristics to allow the children to explore, discover and exploit functional actions like drives. Manipulating these constraints in practice enables inexperienced participants to enhance their physical literacy and motivating them to search for functional actions, without the need to contend with the challenging constraints of the full-scale version of the game. The modified practice environments designed by Fitzpatrick et al. (2017) helped to reduce the immediate challenges of performance constraints, allowing learners to become adept at searching for relevant perception-action couplings, that will eventually be required during performance in the full version of the sport. For example, Fitzpatrick et al. (2017) manipulated essential equipment, such as a tennis ball by reducing its compression, permitting a lower bounce on court, which is better scaled to the dimensions of the forehand and backhand strokes of young children. The lower trajectory of ball flight allowed the children to explore and adopt a swing height that was scaled to their current dimensions as they were growing. These exploratory opportunities in re-scaling actions in practice are useful for the long-term development of their groundstrokes and other skills, compared to the racket swing height needed to strike a regulation tennis ball that bounces higher on court. Evidence suggested that the constraints favoured within mini versions of tennis shape adaptations of movement skills of children during practice. To exemplify, tennis balls with low compression levels positively influenced children's forehand groundstroke performance. Reducing ball compression from 100% (i.e., regulation tennis balls) to 75% has been reported to increase the amount of net-play and elicit a better bounce height for young children learning to hit the ball with groundstrokes, re-scaled to their dimensions. Fitzpatrick and colleagues advocated that the use of modified tennis balls, providing a longer flight phase and lower bounce height due to lower compression, should enable participants to maintain control of longer rallies and in turn facilitating the development of a wider range of strokes. They summarised previous research into the effects of manipulating task constraints, like playing court dimensions and net height, on emergent behaviours of skilled young players. Evidence from research showed that, although average rally length did not differ between conditions, smaller court dimensions elicited fewer winners, and a reduced net height elicited a greater number of winners. The evidence reviewed and provided by Fitzpatrick et al. (2017) suggests how children's physical literacy could be enhanced through opportunities for problem-solving, perception, decision-making and adapting actions by manipulating key task constraints, such as reducing court dimensions and net height. In turn, these changes and the ways that children adapted their actions to them helped to create a relevant psycho-emotional and physical environment for young children to learn to play tennis.

5.6 Attentional Focus

The provision of informational constraints is an important aspect of NLP because they can be useful to guide the exploratory activities of learners at all levels of performance in sport and physical activity. Instructions, as a form of augmented informational constraints can be delivered in different ways to help learners enrich their search and exploration activities (Chow et al., in press; Chow et al., 2016). For example, instructions can be presented to help the learners focus on the *movement form itself* (i.e., how the arms should move or how the trunk should rotate in a throwing action) or the instructions can emphasise the need for accuracy or what the trajectory of a thrown object could look like (e.g., like a rainbow). Different instructions provided to learners can impact learning in different ways. From a NLP perspective, the teacher should consider focusing on the movement outcome rather than the movement form as an over-emphasis on the form can lead to overly conscious control of movements (Chow et al., 2016). Information constraints that emphasise movement form have greater propensity to invoke conscious control of the movement and thus, result in disruption to how the movement could be controlled. According to Bernstein (1967), with increasing sophistication of performance, responsibility for coordination and control is delegated to subordinate levels of the central nervous system (CNS), allowing learners to harness the self-organising movement system dynamics that are most functional for the task. With an external focus of attention, there is little disruption to the lower levels of control as learners are directing their attention to the effect of the movement rather than to the levels of tone or synergies that are critical for movement form itself (see Peh, Chow & Davids, 2011). In learning contexts, if instructions are directed to task specifics, such as how the arms or legs should move, there is greater susceptibility for the control of those movements to be located at a more conscious level of the CNS. This is, however, not to purport that all instructions should then be movement effect oriented. There are indeed some movements where the form is critical and perhaps the use of analogy on how the movement could look like would be relevant (rather than the cues typically prescribing an expected movement form with explicit instructions on the limb movements). Undoubtedly, the use of informational constraints would impact how physical literacy is developed and acquired. Focusing internally could potentially limit the learner's attunement to key perceptual information in the environment that would play a critical role in guiding their actions. Whereas an external focus of attention emphasis could further accentuate the sensitivity of the learner to features in the environment that would encourage more functional movement behaviours (i.e., encouraging direct perception in the skill adaption process).

5.7 Task Simplification

Ensuring strong couplings between information and movement is a key control mechanism espoused in NLP. Specifically, the design principle of **Task Simplification** rather than task decomposition is one important aspect of promoting effective skill acquisition from a NLP perspective (Button et al., 2020; Chow, 2013). Task simplification has clear relevance to the earlier principle of constraints manipulation as the scaling of constraints can allow for greater simplification of a produced movement (this is exemplified by the previous example of scaling playing area dimensions or tennis racket and ball compression properties in mini-tennis games for children: see Fitzpatrick, Davids & Stone, 2018). By incorporating task simplification, learners can develop and maintain strong functional couplings of information that is available to them and the actions that they would generate as a consequence of those information presented in the learning context. In an applied practice context, information is directly perceivable to be picked-up by individual learners to constrain their actions (Chow et al., 2016; Davids et al. 2008). Chow, Davids, Shuttleworth et al. (2020) further suggested that perception is, therefore, a process of searching for the 'specifying' information that can be used to guide the generation of solutions and answers. Undoubtedly, this would have relevance to the earlier pedagogical principle of representativeness in designing practices (Chow et al., in press). Importantly, task simplification provides greater opportunities to achieve success whilst keeping the temporal and spatial challenges of performing the task manageable. Learners have the buffer to move flexibility to explore the environment and generate more information that can be subsequently used for regulating performance (Chow et al., 2016). One example here pertains to how children are challenged to learn how to ride a bike. For little kids, getting onto a balance/pushbike is a great example of task simplification to prepare them to eventually ride a bike with pedals. The locomotion in pushing the bike with alternate limb movements (i.e., running and pushing the bike is a suitable pre-cursor to the actual contra-lateral limb movements for paddling). The need to 'balance' on the bike requires an attunement to subtle adjustments to the bike handle that controls the front wheel to maintain balance. Riding on the balance/pushbike is representative and yet leverages on the principle of task simplification that aids in the acquisition of the movement competency of riding a bike. Task simplification can indeed occur in different ways and the examples given earlier in expanding playing area, incorporating overload conditions in possession games, shortening of rackets (or choking the racket) etc. could be ideas that practitioners may use to trigger more thoughts on how task simplification could be infused in practices.

5.8 Functional Variability

With reference to nonlinearity in learning, variability is seen as inherently present in how movement is controlled and produced. Variability in movement control can thus be functional (Davids et al., 2008). In applied settings, it is desirable that practice variability be incorporated so that the students can be challenged to explore different movement solutions that encourage the close relationship between information and movement to be kept intact (Ranganathan & Newell, 2013). From an Ecological Dynamics perspective, variability is not seen as necessarily undesirable (Chow et al., in press). Rather, variability is critical to allow a system to transit to new behavioural patterns and to move from one functional state to a new functional state (Button et al., 2020; Davids, Bennett & Newell, 2006).

In the context of examining skill adaptation in human movement system, the presence of variability is purported to be an important feature (Hacques et al., 2020). This more functional view of movement variability links well with the need for experience for exploration, search and discovery of task constraints in learners seeking to improve their functional performance in specific contexts. Task constraints manipulation would allow for variability in practice to be enacted. Scaling of task constraints as described earlier and the use of different equipment (e.g., objects with different tactile characteristics) are just some simple examples that variability in practice can be incorporated. However, the introduction of variability should also be undertaken purposefully, with the aim of enriching the experience and performance repertoire of individuals seeking to enhance their physical literacy. It is not just about infusing variability (randomly) in practice contexts. The practitioner should be mindful of how the infused variability in learning could be enriching by directing learners to search differently. Conceptually, the variability in practice can alter the boundaries where learners can search for possible movement solutions and they can be functional or less functional depending on the level of variability incorporated. Overly high levels of variability could potentially lead to random searching and exploration that could be too challenging for some learners, influencing their confidence and motivation. The practitioner must know their sports, games and activity well to understand how the variability can be effectively designed into practices. Nevertheless, variability in practice can be facilitated by effective task constraints manipulation to allow for learners to experience different practice task contexts for a skill to be learnt.

These design principles can then be delivered through the key pedagogical channels of instructions and practices to allow functional goal-directed behaviours to emerge. NLP thus has the potential to provide the design principles and mechanisms that underpin learning activities that are situated in real performance context and suitably catered to the individual learner (Chow, 2013, Chow et al., 2016).

5.9 Exemplifying the Relevance of Nonlinear Pedagogy in Practice: The 'Why' Question

Most of the previous work that examined the efficacy of NLP was based on recent findings from the motor control and learning literature that highlighted how the human movement system behaves like a nonlinear system and how learning as well as teaching processes captures these key traits of a nonlinear system (Chow, 2013). Our own work with teachers and students in schools and studies by Lee et al. (2014) and Lee et al. (2017) in formal educational settings have provided valuable insights into the relevance of NLP in supporting teaching and learning. Lee et al. (2014) investigated students from a Singapore primary school with no tennis background who underwent a learning intervention over several weeks comprising either the NLP or Linear Pedagogy (LP) condition (i.e., a traditional pedagogical approach with an emphasis on drill and technique commonly present in physical education context). Changes in performance were observed at three levels: (1) the individual; (2) in a game setting and (3) in a class setting. Findings showed that the students in the NLP condition were just as effective as the LP condition even though they received less explicit prescriptive instructions on movement form in the former condition. These findings suggest that perhaps there is more than one functional way to solve our movement challenges – many ways of moving to achieve the same target – evidence of *degenerate* behaviours where there could be many movement pathways to achieve the same outcome (Rein, Davids & Button, 2009; Seifert et al., 2016). Without a doubt, system degeneracy is intimately linked to enhanced levels of physical literacy. Specifically, it would indicate that if learners have meaningfully developed their physical literacy, transfer and adaptation to various performance environment would be easier and more relevant. Indeed, this has implications on how talent can be developed and how there could be the presence of donor sports to support specialised participation in elite sports eventually.

In the same study by Lee et al. (2014), it was also found that the LP group had difficulty retaining the movement behaviours that were taught to them where the emphasis was on the prescriptive expected movement form for the tennis stroke. There was a tendency for the students to revert to movement patterns that were more individualised and different to the prescribed movements. Critically, whilst it was anticipated that the LP approach with a focus on direct explicit instructions would be more effective, it did not pan out as typically expected. These are insightful findings as the results suggest that students can engage in exploratory behaviours and acquire more individualised movement solutions to achieve success where the emphasis is on the students (i.e., student focused).

In another study by Lee et al. (2017) where NLP was examined in its efficacy in encouraging the acquisition of 21st century competencies, it was found that NLP encouraged teachers to create representative learning designs through the inclusion of a variety of modified games which allowed for greater freedom for the students to direct their own learning. There was an emphasis on exploration and problem-solving which can be relevant to supporting the students to develop 21st century competencies. The key findings in Lee et al. (2017), based on qualitative interviews of students and teachers, provided insights on how NLP created a learning environment that potentially facilitated perceived competence, autonomy and relatedness which could enhance intrinsic motivation and enjoyment for the students during their physical education lessons. In a subsequent chapter, case studies will be shared to discuss the impact of NLP on learners' motivation to be engaged in physical activity and thus instrumental in encouraging the development of physical literacy.

In a more recent work by Chow et al. (2019), it was reported that a NLP intervention was just as effective as a LP intervention for a territorial game and in the teaching and learning of fundamental movement skills. It was found that students presented with a NLP approach had different learning experiences (e.g., more opportunities for collaboration, less pressured to follow an optimal expected movement behaviour) and this was similar to the findings of Lee et al. (2014). Importantly, interview data collected with the teachers, provided important insights into how teachers' behaviours could potentially be shaped when the focus is on encouraging exploratory behaviours by the students.

In the work related to examining the impact of NLP on the adaptation of fundamental movement skills by children in two Singapore schools, it was found that students who were presented with a NLP intervention (lasting eight weeks during the PE lessons) were at least as good as those in the LP condition or better (Chow et al., 2019) based on data from TGMD-2 results. The students in the NLP condition achieved higher scores for running and stationary dribbling at a post-test session, as well as elevation of scores for the overhand throw between post- and pre-test sessions. Referencing the Validated Developmental Sequences (Goodway, Ozmun & Gallahue, 2019), it was also determined that there was a greater transition in terms of percentage of students from Elementary Stage to Mature

Stage for the skills of sliding and stationary dribble from pre- to post- test for NLP condition group as compared to LP condition group. Further interview data of both students and teachers also found that the learning processes differed qualitatively between NLP and LP conditions. Students presented with the NLP intervention demonstrated behaviours that showed greater exploration in their learning (i.e., trying different movement solutions in representative learning tasks that are not too prescriptive). Nevertheless, some of the teachers involved in the study responded that, whilst NLP seemed to encourage more active learning on the part of the students, some form of inclusion of LP type instructions may still be relevant (i.e., consider an NLP-LP hybrid approach). In brief, findings from Chow et al. (2019) showed promising results for NLP and more of such empirical studies could be conducted in the schools.

Komar et al. (2014), in a pedagogical setting, showed that in early practice, merely practising breaststroke without any pedagogical support led to an improvement in performance after two months. Moreover, this improvement in performance was not different compared to another group that received instructions about how to swim more efficiently (i.e., more prescriptive information). The intervention group received instructions that were analogy-based and specifically without any prescription of an ideal technique to follow (aligned to the principles of NLP). Whilst it was observed that performance in the control group did improve, it was ascertained that the performance improvement was due to an optimisation of the initial behaviour instead of the adoption of a more efficient one (i.e., they improved because there was room for significant enhancement and not due to the acquisition of a more functional and effective movement behaviour eventually). As highlighted by Komar et al. (2014), there is a suggestion that the swimmers in the control group may have increased their force impulse during arm or leg propulsion in order to counteract the higher water resistances due to their inefficient movements. In the case of the intervention group provided with NLP, the effectiveness of NLP manifested itself through the adoption of an efficient movement behaviour and this would logically be an anticipated progression for the acquisition of higher expert mastery (i.e., skill stage of learning) as the learners engage in more practice over time (see Newell, 1986).

Whilst there is a need for more research in practical settings, such as formal learning contexts, the findings from the current body of empirical studies indicate great potential for NLP to work effectively to support teaching, coaching and learning. Clearly, the implications to practitioners and policymakers include how we should question the traditional one-size-fits-all, outcome-based philosophy that has dominated PE and sports historically. Consider how learning experiences should be enriching and how it develops throughout the lifespan, focusing on recreation and general skill adaptation earlier in life and then seek opportunities for specialisation later when engaged in high-performance sports (Stone et al., 2018; Strafford et al., 2018). It is time to rethink teacher and coach education; review professional development for physical education teachers and coaches and importantly, reconsider how we may even conduct assessment with reference to physical literacy.

5.10 How Can Nonlinear Pedagogy Be Applied to Enhance Physical Literacy?

Concepts in NLP may be perceived as challenging to understand and perhaps even more so with reference to enacting it in practical settings. Yet strangely, some practitioners may already be using some of the design principles underpinning NLP. For example,

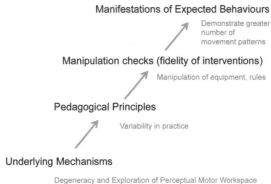

FIGURE 5.2 Degeneracy and exploration of perceptual motor workspace

practitioners would have on numerous occasions manipulated task constraints in the form of information or equipment in their practice sessions to promote the attainment of physical literacy.

Nevertheless, the 'how' of NLP is an important aspect that practitioners are keen to understand and apply. It should be noted that NLP does not mandate the use of all design principles for all contexts. It is not a framework that provides a formula where practitioners have to religiously use in some sequence to ensure that the NLP approach is to be effectively delivered. It is not meant only for sports and games. In all skill acquisition and adaptation contexts where the enhancement of physical literacy is the goal, NLP could be applicable and not all design principles have to be used at the same time. The purpose of the design principles captured in NLP is to provide a framework to see how these principles are underpinned by concepts in Ecological Dynamics that has direct relevance to motor control mechanisms in supporting the development of physical literacy. To elucidate the couplings between practice tasks, manipulation checks, design principles and control mechanisms, please refer to the Figure 5.2.

The design pedagogical principles in NLP must be relevant to motor learning mechanisms. For example, infusing variability in practice harnesses inherent degeneracy in the human neurobiological system and allows for exploratory behaviours to surface, be discovered and exploited. Infusion of variability in practice can be enacted through the thoughtful (i.e., non-random) manipulation of task constraints (ensuring fidelity of interventions that variability is indeed increased) such as the use of equipment or changing playing space or rules of the learning task (e.g., throwing to different directions, inclusion of opponents or providing asymmetrically designed playgrounds). If the intervention of increasing variability is effective, there should be some expected manifestations of behaviours such as learners demonstrating greater movement patterns with reference to the task. Such an understanding of the relevance between control mechanisms, pedagogical principles, manipulation checks and the manifestations of expected behaviours provides practitioners with greater clarity on how practices can be designed to effectively promote NLP.

Similarly, manipulation of constraints is underpinned by the concept of parametric control where constraints can be scaled to push a learner's movement system to transit between stable patterns of behaviours. Representativeness is relevant to notions of adaptability and transferability. Task simplification is aligned to the ideas of ensuring information-movement couplings despite changes to how the task dynamics may alter.

In a sample lesson plan (see Table 5.1) on catching (a ball), the activities are designed according to the relevant design pedagogical principles for NLP. Each of the principles is related to the control mechanisms as seen in the last column of the sample lesson plan. The teaching cues/instructions and use of suggested equipment are akin to the manipulation checks to ensure fidelity of the planned interventions. In this case, learners could demonstrate different catching behaviours (as a manifestation of expected behaviours).

In a recent piece of work to exemplify how NLP could be applicable for young children learning fundamental movement skills, Chow, Davids, Renshaw et al. (2020) described a series of learning activities underpinned by NLP design principles. NLP could be used in a gymnastic lesson with young children, to focus on enrichment of physical literacy through rolling and highlighting its different pedagogical principles.

In Chow, Davids, Renshaw, et al. (2020), it was highlighted how infusing **representativeness** could be useful in especially designing learning environment for young children where enjoyment and fun is paramount. Using imaginative storytelling, gymnastics lessons can be situated in the context of storybooks and one example given was *The Gruffalo*, a popular story that many children would be familiar with. This children's book tells the story of a small mouse who encounters and outwits a host of predators in a deep dark wood. Incorporating *The Gruffalo* into gymnastics lessons can be used to create a whole range of affordances that children can exploit in the learning environment. Children can adopt different characters from the book and move in ways that they think the characters would move. For example, in a lesson on rolling, the children can see themselves as the 'snake' in the story and this analogy could provide the children with opportunities to move their bodies close to the floor and over and under equipment (like the snake!).

The **manipulation of constraints** in the rolling gymnastics lesson could also facilitate children to innovatively move around the play space like characters from *The Gruffalo*. The use of equipment like benches, horses and mats together with the play space available affords different opportunities for the children to explore movements like in a playground. These movements could again be pegged to how the different characters in *The Gruffalo* might move. The dynamic interaction between the performer, task and environment constraints affords possibilities for the children to explore moving in different ways. In this scenario practitioners have the autonomy to design and create different settings for the children. For example, if a child tends to repeat the same movement solutions consistently whilst travelling around the play space, he/she could be encouraged to move out of his/her comfort zone and be challenged to adapt by reading further into the book and introducing one of the predators into the play space (see Chow, Davids, Renshaw, et al., 2020). The inclusion of a game of tag (change of task constraints in terms of rules) would also invite different actions on the part of the children. This could infuse some form of instability (i.e., competitive play instead of cooperative play) that would channel the children to find and move into space so as to avoid other children.

Movement creates information that can be directly perceived and in turn supports further movement in a cyclical process (i.e., information-movement coupling). This information-movement coupling is maintained within gymnastics lessons by having all large equipment (gym mats, wedges, wall bars) present throughout the duration of each lesson. The key factor is to consider manipulating constraints to allow for **task simplification** that keeps the temporal and spatial challenges manageable for the children. For example, using smaller obstacles on the floor to encourage jumping or hopping over it, using bars that allow for easier grips to challenge the children to hang on to it in a swinging action. This

TABLE 5.1 Exemplar from simple Nonlinear Pedagogy plan

Lesson time	Nonlinear pedagogy – Lesson	Objectives			
		Perform a catch			
Time	Activity	Teaching cues/Instructions Cues and Instructions	Organisation/Equipment	Pedagogical Principles	Mechanisms
10 mins	**Catch Everything** • Cooperative activity where students work in pairs. A tosses a 'ball' and B catches the ball. • B then tosses back to A to catch. Go for 5 consecutive catches. Challenge students by increasing number of consecutive passes. • Change type of balls used by having different "ball" on each station. 'Balls' placed in a basket. • Get students to try out different passes. Besides tossing, can attempt a bounce pass to partner for certain types of balls. • Consider having an 'opponent' between the pair as a progression (simulate a defender) • Consider positioning a net or a rope between the pair (as an alternative barrier)	• Students to explore as many ways to catch successfully when catching different types of balls • Imagine your hands are like a net • Imagine the hands are like a cushion when you catch the object	• Basketball • Tennis ball • Rolled-up towels/t-shirts • Rolled-up socks • Bean bag • Objects to be throw can be left within a hula hoop	• Manipulation of constraints • Functional variability • Representative learning design • Task simplification	• Parametric control • Degeneracy • Transferability • Information-movement coupling

can be done in the absence of explicit prescriptive instructions. Practitioners can design the learning environment to create opportunities for children to search and exploit self-organisation tendencies (i.e., emergence of behaviours as a consequence of the interactions amongst constraints), leading to better spatial awareness and being more in tune socially with their peers over time (Chow, Davids, Renshaw, et al., 2020). The practitioner should see themselves as designer of practices and consider the importance of helping the children to establish meaningful information-movement couplings through activities that promotes creativity and experimentation on the part of the children. Movements can then be learned in context, and skills need not be isolated and developed by separating them into components (Chow, Davids, Renshaw, et al., 2020).

For young children, it would be very useful for imaginative mini-games to be designed into lessons with analogies and questions. Activities can be incorporated to create an external **focus of attention** and opportunities for problem-solving which require functional movement solutions from each child, without the requirement of explicit instructions from the practitioner (Chow, Davids, Renshaw, et al., 2020). An example is a gymnastics lesson, which can involve a game where the children could role play as a snake who must move treasure (beanbags) from one side of the water (their mat) to the other. The treasure must not get wet and each bit of treasure must be moved across the water in different ways to avoid the attention of *The Gruffalo* (see Chow, Davids, Renshaw, et al., 2020). There is no specific prescription on how the children should move since each child may imagine themselves differently in the way they could move. Such activities really accentuate the joy of being involved in active play.

There could be occasions when some children may be seen as being stuck in a rut and not be making much progress. Infusion of **variability in practice** could be needed to help the children explore new movements that could get them out of the rut and to something more functional. For example, in the snake game played in the gymnastics rolling lesson, instability through movement variability can be created by giving children different types of equipment (treasure) to transport (i.e., of different sizes, shapes or weights) across the mat (which can also vary in dimensions) (see Chow, Davids, Renshaw, et al., 2020). Critically, when variability is added into the practice, changing task constraints can result in new affordances being available, providing children with the opportunities to interact with the task and environment that could result in creative and innovative ways to move.

We will revisit this example of using a popular story (like *The Gruffalo*) to situate learning experiences for children to engage in physical activities and how it would potentially help develop their physical literacy. These foundational movement skills that the children learn may help to build a transferable foundation for further engagement in specialised sports and games. This is aligned to the other major pedagogical approach shared in this book, Athletic Skills Model (ASM), in terms of its relevance to develop talent and physical literacy. The ASM is a pedagogical framework that offers an alternative programme structure that evolved from professional sports practice and proposes the importance of the role that a diverse range of sport experiences can enhance and enrich later specialisation in sport (Wormhoudt et al., 2017) (more in-depth discussion on ASM would be undertaken in subsequent chapters). Importantly, meaningful engagement by children involved in such learning experiences can lead to increased motivation to participate in physical activities and several case studies in the later chapters of this book will help to exemplify the impact of NLP on the affective domain in PE and sports.

To conclude this chapter, the use of NLP provides an exciting platform to enhance physical literacy for learners. It takes into account the learner-environment mutuality, underpinned by design principles that promote exploration for the individual. The what, why and how of NLP could be a useful frame for practitioners to better understand children's movements in teaching and learning contexts. In the subsequent chapters, we will continue to build on the narrative of how NLP (and ASM) can be strong cornerstones to help our children and young adults to develop physical literacy that would provide meaningful engagement in physical activity throughout a person's lifespan.

References

Adolph, K. E. & Hoch, J. E. (2019). Motor development: Embodied, embedded, enculturated, and enabling. *Annual Review of Psychology*, *70*, 141–164.

Bernstein, N. A. (1967). *The co-ordination and regulation of movements*. Oxford: Pergamon Press.

Button, C., Lee, C. Y., Dutt-Mazumder, A., Tan, W. K. & Chow, J. Y. (2012). Empirical investigations of nonlinear motor learning. *The Open Sports Sciences Journal*, *5*(Suppl 1-M6), 49–58. doi:10.2174/1875399X01205010049.

Button, C., Seifert, L., Chow, J. Y., Araújo, D. & Davids, K. (2020). *Dynamics of skill acquisition: an ecological dynamics approach* (Second ed.). Champaign, IL: Human Kinetics Publishers.

Chow, J. Y. (2013). Nonlinear learning underpinning pedagogy: Evidence, challenges and implications. *Quest*, *65*, 469–484. doi:10.1080/00336297.2013.807746.

Chow, J. Y., Davids, K., Button, C. & Renshaw, I. (2016). *Nonlinear pedagogy in skill acquisition: An introduction*. New York: Routledge.

Chow, J. Y., Davids, K., Hristovski, R., Araújo, D. & Passos, P. (2011). Nonlinear pedagogy: Learning design for self-organizing neurobiological systems. *New Ideas in Psychology*, *29*(2), 189–200.

Chow, J. Y., Davids, K., Renshaw, I. & Rudd, J. (2020). Nonlinear pedagogy. In M. A. Peters & R. Heraud (Eds.), *Encyclopedia of educational innovation* (pp. 1–7). Singapore: Springer.

Chow, J. Y., Davids, K., Shuttleworth, R. & Araújo, D. (2020). Ecological dynamics and transfer from practice to performance in sport. In N. Hodges & M. Williams (Eds.), *Skill acquisition in sport* (pp. 330–344). London: Routledge.

Chow, J. Y., Komar, J., Davids, K. & Tan, C. W. K. (in press). Nonlinear Pedagogy and its implications for practice in the Singapore PE context. *Physical Education and Sport Pedagogy*.

Chow, J. Y., Renshaw, I., Button, C., Davids, K. & Tan, C. W. K. (2013). Effective learning design for the individual: A nonlinear pedagogical approach in physical education. In A. Ovens, T. Hopper & J. Butler (Eds.), *Complexity thinking in physical education: Reframing curriculum, pedagogy and research* (pp. 121–134). London: Routledge.

Chow, J. Y., Teo-Koh, S. M., Tan, W. K. C., Tan, S. J. B., Button, C. M. R., Kapur, M. & Choo, Z. Y. C. (2019). *Nonlinear pedagogy and its relevance for the New PE curriculum* (NIE Research Brief Series No. 19-012). Singapore: National Institute of Education.

Correia, V., Carvalho, J., Araújo, D., Pereira, E. & Davids, K. (2019). Principles of nonlinear pedagogy in sport practice. *Physical Education and Sport Pedagogy*, *24*(2), 117–132.

Davids, K., Bennett, S. & Newell, K. M. (2006). *Movement system variability*. Champaign, IL: Human kinetics.

Fitzpatrick, A., Davids, K. & Stone, J. A. (2017). Effects of lawn tennis association mini tennis as task constraints on children's match-play characteristics. *Journal of Sports Sciences*, *35*(22), 2204–2210.

Fitzpatrick, A., Davids, K. & Stone, J. A. (2018). Effects of scaling task constraints on emergent behaviours in children's racquet sports performance. *Human Movement Science*, *58*, 80–87.

Goodway, J. D., Ozmun, J. C. & Gallahue, D. L. (2019). *Understanding motor development: Infants, children, adolescents, adults*. Burlington, VT: Jones & Bartlett Learning.

Hacques, G., Komar, J., Dicks, M. & Seifert, L. (2020). Exploring to learn and learning to explore. *Psychological Research*, 10.1007/s00426-020-01352-x. Advance online publication. https://doi.org/10.1007/s00426-020-01352-x

Henry, F. M. (1958). Specificity vs generality in learning motor skills. *Proc Coll Phys Educ Assoc. 61,* 126–128.

Komar, J., Chow, J. Y., Chollet, D. & Seifert, L. (2014). Effect of analogy instructions with an internal focus on learning a complex motor skill. *Journal of Applied Sport Psychology, 26*(1), 17–32.

Lee, M. C. Y., Chow, J. Y., Button, C. & Tan, C. W. K. (2017). Nonlinear pedagogy and its role in encouraging twenty-first century competencies through physical education: A Singapore experience. *Asia Pacific Journal of Education, 37*(4), 483–499. doi:10.1080/02188791.2017.1386089.

Lee, M. C. Y., Chow, J. Y., Komar, J., Tan, C. W. K. & Button, C. (2014). Nonlinear pedagogy: An effective approach for novices to learn sports skills. *PLoS ONE, 9*(8), e104744.

Newell, K. (1986). Constraints on the development of coordination. In M. G. Wade & H. T. A. Whiting (Eds.), Motor development in children: Aspects of coordination and control (pp. 341–360). The Netherlands: Springer.

Orth, D., van der Kamp, J. & Button, C. (2019). Learning to be adaptive as a distributed process across the coach–athlete system: Situating the coach in the constraints-led approach. *Physical Education and Sport Pedagogy, 24*(2), 146–161.

Ovens, A., Hopper, T. & Butler, J. (Eds.). (2013). *Complexity thinking in physical education: Reframing curriculum, pedagogy, and research.* London: Routledge.

Peh, S. Y. C., Chow, J. Y. & Davids, K. (2011). Focus of attention and its impact on movement behaviour. *Journal of Science and Medicine in Sport, 14*(1), 70–78.

Pinder, R. A. & Renshaw, I. (2019). What can coaches and physical education teachers learn from a constraints-led approach in para-sport? *Physical Education and Sport Pedagogy, 24*(2), 190–205.

Ranganathan, R. & Newell, K. M. (2013). Changing up the routine: Intervention-induced variability in motor learning. *Exercise and Sport Sciences Reviews, 41*(1), 64–70.

Rein, R., Davids, K. & Button, C. (2009). Adaptive and phase transition behavior in performance of discrete multi-articular actions by degenerate neurobiological systems. *Experimental Brain Research, 201*(2), 307–322. doi:10.1007/s00221-009-2040-x.

Renshaw, I. & Chow, J. Y. (2019). A constraint-led approach to sport and physical education pedagogy. *Physical Education and Sport Pedagogy, 24*(2), 103–116. doi:10.1080/17408989.2018.1552676.

Roberts, W. M., Newcombe, D. J. & Davids, K. (2019). Application of a constraints-led approach to pedagogy in schools: Embarking on a journey to nurture physical literacy in primary physical education. *Physical Education and Sport Pedagogy, 24*(2), 162–175.

Seifert, L., Komar, J., Araújo, D. & Davids, K. (2016). Neurobiological degeneracy: A key property for functional adaptations of perception and action to constraints. *Neuroscience and Biobehavioral Reviews, 69*, 159–65. doi:10.1016/j.neubiorev.2016.08.006.

Stone, J. A., Strafford, B. W., North, J. S., Toner, C. & Davids, K. (2018). Effectiveness and efficiency of virtual reality designs to enhance athlete development: An ecological dynamics perspective. *Movement & Sport Sciences-Science & Motricité,* (102), 51–60. doi: 10.1051/sm/2018031.

Strafford, B. W., Van Der Steen, P., Davids, K. & Stone, J. A. (2018). Parkour as a donor sport for athletic development in youth team sports: Insights through an ecological dynamics lens. *Sports Medicine-Open, 4*(1), 21.

Wormhoudt, R., Savelsbergh, G. J., Teunissen, J. W. & Davids, K. (2017). The athletic skills model: Optimizing talent development through movement education. London: Routledge.

6

PRACTITIONERS AS ARCHITECTS OF THE ENVIRONMENT

How We Can Use Environmental Design Principles to Support Physical Literacy

Danny Newcombe, Keith Davids and Will Roberts

6.1 Environment Architects to Support Physical Literacy

The manipulation (alteration, adaptation, refinement) of task constraints is an important role for practitioners who may be considered learning designers or architects of learning environments. It is important at this point to emphasise the key role that practitioners play in designing innovative and robust tasks, sessions, programmes and curricula which facilitate transferable and targeted development for learners. Recently, we have argued that the role of the practitioner as environment architect must be given greater emphasis (Renshaw et al., 2019). This role is driven by an under-appreciation of how nuanced the successful application of the principles of Nonlinear Pedagogy needs to be in the creation, and delivery, of effective programmes and their associated practice environments. As illustrated in earlier chapters, the challenge for practitioners is to provide carefully designed environments that make available a wide range of desired affordances that will enhance an individual's capacities to discover, explore and exploit surrounding information from the environment to continually search for solutions as they reorganise and exploit the way that parts of the body are coordinated, a task that is much easier said than done. The specific focus for a practitioner (teacher or coach) should be to view themselves as a problem setter, one who designs a curriculum of activities that allow individuals or groups of individuals (i.e., functioning in teams) to self-organise and co-adapt to achieve the goal-directed behaviour, or simply put, effectively solve the problem set by the practitioner.

6.2 Guiding Frameworks

The key challenge for practitioners in physical education, sport and play concerns how to operationalise in practice an understanding of physical literacy as viewed through children's *functional movement skill* (see Chapter 2). As highlighted in Chapter 1, there is a need to move towards more 'unstructured' children's play-based activities that can enrich relevant behaviours that are vital for human development. The development of these valuable skills and abilities impact on each individual's capacity to negotiate play and performance contexts in the future, adapting their actions to the environmental constraints that they encounter. We have emphasised the significant role that practitioners play in the creation of effective practice environments and have proposed that practitioners should see themselves as environment architects when designing sessions, programmes and curricula. However, integrating theoretical ideas into practical learning design can be challenging, as employing new ideas in practice can be a daunting and confusing task. It is this gap, between the theoretical underpinnings of physical literacy and practical applications, that is often cited as the most significant barrier practitioners face as they negotiate the pragmatics of learning design (Greenwood, Davids & Renshaw, 2014). In a recent commentary paper, we called for the provision of *frameworks* to support practitioners in a robust environment design process (Newcombe et al., 2019). These frameworks are positioned to support integration of theoretical understanding and its practical application. They have the potential to act as a guidance tool for practitioners to ensure they are designing environments consistent with the nurturing physical literacy in learners. The provision of frameworks, underpinned by understanding of the development of physical literacy as an embedded and embodied process, will support a more nuanced application, enabling practitioners to make more accurate and informed design decisions in learning environments. In the following sections we will bring the process of curriculum and learning design to life as we explore how frameworks can be employed to guide the creation of a programme curriculum.

6.3 Programme Landscapes

It is important to appreciate that educators across all movement discourses (physical educators, sports coaches and physiotherapists) are designing programmes across multiple timescales of performance, learning and development, in an effort to enhance the skills and capabilities of children and athletes in their care (Woods, Rudd, et al., 2020). From a design perspective, one of the greatest challenges for practitioners, regardless of context (across a continuum from physical education to high-performance sport), is to develop programmes that, rather than being episodic in nature, are connected and have continuity across performance, learning and development, thereby supporting physical literacy. The learner and practitioner enter into an appreciation of wayfinding and a shared ethos of representative co-design (Woods, Rothwell, et al., 2020). In doing so, they move away from a traditional, hierarchical model of the learner-practitioner relationship, often characterised by mechanistic perspectives of the learning process, which Bernstein (1967), p. 234) decried as 'mechanical repetition by rote'. This traditional and hierarchical model often places the practitioner at the core of the instructional process, providing the learner with instructions for reproducing a technique, as well as prescribing sequentially corrective feedback for continued reproduction and compliance. This traditional approach is synonymous to a navigational device indicating that an adaptation to a journey is a 'wrong' turn that deviates from the prescribed 'best' or 'fastest' route. By situating the learner at the core of practice design, a practitioner can design a landscape that invites a learner to explore and exploit available affordances during the learning process. In this sense, there would be no 'wrong' turns, just opportunities for learners to continually explore system degeneracy in a variety of potential destination 'routes' within the confines of the landscape designed. Learners would be free to settle on a particular 'route' they feel suffices their intentions, action capabilities and environmental constraints. An example of such an approach in high-performance sport could involve the coach designing a practice task that encourages particularly difficult or more creative passes between teammates in team sports like basketball, rugby union or football, inviting learners to explore and experience different ways of performing them. An example of how an understanding of the Environment Design Principles (EDP) can be employed to help to meet this intention is provided by exploring and employing the *repetition without repetition* principle, one of its core practice design principles (Renshaw et al., 2019). By manipulating task constraints in order to design-in the appropriate amount of (in)stability and variability to the practice task we create the need and the opportunity for learners to perceive and utilise the affordances available to perform the action in a more creative manner. However, providing an appropriate level of (in)stability and variability for a group of learners, all of whom have unique intrinsic dynamics (a set of skills, dispositions, playing history, wants and needs), is a challenge for practitioners that should not be underestimated. In the following sections we introduce the EDP, positioning them as bridge between theoretical concepts that underpin Nonlinear Pedagogy and its practical application.

6.4 The Environment Design Principles

The aim of this section is to familiarise the reader with the EDP (Renshaw et al., 2019). The EDP consist of four key principles that capture the core theoretical foundations of a Nonlinear Pedagogy. The key principles are: (1) Session Aim, (2) Constrain to afford, (3) Representative learning design and (4) Repetition without repetition (which is framed around manipulating variability to enhance adaptability and increase or decrease (in)stability). Each principle has its own unique purpose, resultantly impacting upon decisions a coach will make in the curriculum design process. It is through the integration of all four principles that the framework is able to operate effectively and efficiently. In this way, the EDP look to support practitioner decision-making, as the teacher or coach engages in the messy process of learning design. We introduce and explain each principle throughout this chapter by exploring how they interact with development of physical literacy.

6.4.1 Targeted Development

Principle 1 emphasises the role and importance targeted development in the curriculum design process. First, we pose the question: 'does our sport session, physical education lesson, play activity educate the learner about their world?' This question signifies that practitioners need to recognise, and take into consideration, that participants are situated in an ecological niche (i.e., including the home environment, club, school, athlete training camp). These contexts have access to particular spaces (garden, park, playground, field or specialist equipment). This is the 'performance' landscape that learners are currently (self) navigating to find their path, shaping their ongoing physical literacy.

Next, the aim of the session is an integral driver of the coach or teacher's decision-making as they plan their curriculum, prepare and design their practice environments. In a previous book, we were advocating these ideas at a session level, but it is equally important at a more global level. It is important that we have a clear area of targeted development for the block, programme or season (or cycle) of sessions. The importance of having overarching aims and understanding the impact they have on the designed interactions between learners and the landscape of affordances has been introduced and explored in previous literature (Renshaw et al., 2019). Over-arching aims could include, for example: (i) enrichment of underlying physical, psychological, emotional and social capacities by providing opportunities for learners to explore their environment and successfully adapt their actions to changing constraints; (ii) enhanced coordination of actions of a group of learners; (iii) confidence to undertake novel, innovative and creative actions, in response to music and rhythms and (iv) problem-solving capacities to understand how a task has changed due to different circumstances and (re)organise actions accordingly. As environment designers we need to appreciate that our focus or chosen area of targeted development not only impacts on our decision-making as teachers/coaches, but can act as an over-riding constraint (individual) on performer(s), influencing their use of cognitions, perceptions and actions within a play/practice environment. In Chapter 2 we highlighted the importance of *individual intentions* in the emergent *wayfinding* process and developing a deep knowledge of the environment. Therefore, as a practitioner engages in the curriculum design process, it is critical that they establish the primary goal(s) of the practice block as a first step, this will then in-turn shape the design of the specific practice environments employed to achieve the overarching aim (in individual session tasks). As previously alluded to, the unique nature of every context requires that various elements of learning tasks can be added, removed, adjusted or repositioned within the curriculum to bring about the desired intention(s). This task constraints manipulation process is both complex and nuanced, requiring careful consideration, governed by the intention.

> **Reflection** – *As practitioners we have previously fallen into the trap of providing generic environments that lack specific purpose and any form of targeted development. We have found that investing time at the start of the design process, establishing the key aims within our curriculum provides us with the guiding light we need to design an effective curriculum.*

The goal(s) of a training block and associated practice environments can, and should, vary considerably for practitioners and learners. For example, one of the development themes could be to develop a new skill set in the learners (e.g., navigating space by single-leg hoping). We may decide that the learners need to increase their repertoire of options by which they can pass a basketball, with a specific technical focus of keeping the ball trajectory flat and hard. Or we may want to encourage the defenders to explore new tackling methods with the aim of winning the ball back within a soccer context. Alternatively, it may be the aim of the teaching team to help learners to collaborate together, understanding how they can co-adapt their decisions and actions when searching for tactical solutions. Figure 6.1

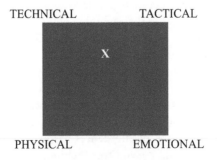

FIGURE 6.1 Technical, tactical, emotional and physical session intention locator tool

provides a tool designed to help the coach or teacher to consider the development area we are looking to focus on. Within our play-based environment we often ask the question: 'what are we turning the volume up on today?'. Whilst all four elements will always be incorporated within any of our practice environments, the consideration of where the 'X' is located encourages us to be clearer on what we want to dial up within the session or practice. One of our challenges is managing many competing development needs with limited contact time. Ultimately, it helps to guide what we prioritise and the decisions we make around the types of practice we employ and how they are adjusted to meet the groups intention(s).

> **Reflection** – *As a curriculum design team we have often attempted to focus on multiple aims concurrently. Unfortunately, this approach has manifested itself with the provision of generic sessions and diluted practices that are trying to do too much and, therefore, less likely to have any targeted impact on a group or individual level. We find it is best to have one single clear intention that underpinned each game, and this provided a clear direction for the design and delivery process.*

When the primary goal of the session is to promote learning, the practice environments need to be designed to allow learners the opportunity to *explore*, *exploit* or *execute* solutions. Figure 6.2 provides us with an additional intention locator tool, again promoting a consideration of whether the focus of the session is for the learners to explore, exploit, or execute new solutions, perhaps to a technical or tactical problem we have set. As with the previous locator, we can use this tool to guide the decisions we make as we design and adjust our practice environments. For a detailed example of how these tools are operationalised in practice, we direct you to the performance hockey case study, located in Chapter 12.

As previously alluded to, practitioners need to appreciate that session intention (or targeted development) act as an over-riding constraint on performer and team cognitions, perceptions and actions. In considering our targeted development, there must also be an alignment between the intentions of the coach and the intentions of the athletes(s). A disparity between a performer's intentions and a coach or teacher's desired actions can lead to failure and ultimately frustration for both the coach and the performer(s).

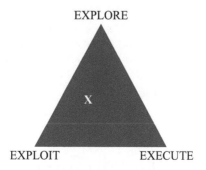

FIGURE 6.2 Explore, exploit and execute session intention locator tool

6.4.2 *Constrain to Afford*

In Chapter 2, we presented Ecological Dynamics as a framework to develop understanding of *functional movement skills* and how this is at the heart of physical literacy. In this section we will build on this information by providing examples of how practitioners can use this principle to create and structure enriched environments to support and cultivate a life-long affinity for physical activity (Rudd et al., 2020; O'Sullivan et al., 2020). Ecological Dynamics provides a characterisation of learning as the development of a child's ability to perceive information and self-organise under constraints, exploiting the affordances that exist within the performance landscape emphasises the importance of practitioners being able to employ the 'constrain to afford' principle.

The ability to 'design-in' constraints to invite learners to explore effective solutions related to the session aim is core to the *constrain to afford* principle. The principle brings together two important concepts located within Nonlinear Pedagogic framework that is relevant for the enrichment of physical literacy in learners: constraints and affordances. The challenge for practitioners is to manipulate relevant constraints as they systematically design-in opportunities to use available affordances to the practice environment. To achieve this aim, the value and meaning of affordances need to be learned by individuals. In essence practitioners could view themselves as problem setters who design practice tasks to facilitate targeted, implicit skill development. Whilst all practice environments present a problem for learners to solve, the practitioner's role is to adjust and adapt the problems set, ensuring that task designs present a specific problem associated with the session aim. We have termed not doing enough to manipulate key task constraints in the practice environment: '*under constraining*'. Skill learning in this context is predicated on children learning to adapt to the environment through the process of attunement to, and exploitation of, key affordances in the landscape. It is therefore a requirement of a curriculum to foster physical literacy to provide practice environments that specifically offer opportunities for performers to become more attuned and develop the ability to effectively interact with the affordances present in the performance environment (Araújo & Davids, 2011). A key challenge for practitioners is to manipulate constraints in order to emphasise or exaggerate the availability of relevant affordances. This process aims to direct learners' search within a performance environment, promoting the ability of individuals to 'pick up' and effectively interact with the key affordances effectively. This process is called *Constraining to Afford*. As *learning designers*, practitioners can manipulate constraints that will educate the attention of learners to perceive and utilise available affordances within a practice task. To clarify, practitioners do not design affordances. In their work they should design learning tasks that help learners to perceive and utilise available affordances, channelling individuals towards their availability in the landscape (Chow et al., 2016). In the following section we provide an outline of the three-step process of *offer, invite* and apply *co-adaptation*, which underpins learning design. In the curriculum design section that follows we present examples of this principle in action, focusing on how these concepts guide the decisions that practitioners can take during the development of practice tasks.

6.4.2.1 *Offer Key Affordances*

Step 1 challenges coaches and teachers to build an environment that provides learners with the opportunity to engage with the information and affordances available related to the development focus (session aim). By using knowledge about human movement and inter-acting systems, it is the role of the practitioner to facilitate these opportunities for action through the manipulation of key *task* constraints. For example, if we want learners to develop their understanding of how far they can hop and control their landing, by spread-ing out flat markers randomly in the performance landscape, we can offer the learners the challenge of hopping and landing over varied distances.

6.4.2.2 Invite and Encourage Interaction with Key Affordances

Step 2 involves manipulating the constraints of the practice environment to encourage individuals to engage with important affordances in an effective and efficient manner as they self-organise and attempt to solve the problem presented. Essentially, moving past step 1, where we just provide the opportunity to hop and stick. For example, if we inte-grate a 1v1 evasion game and/or add in a drum beat into the hopping landscape we encour-age learners to explore how far they can hop and stick in order to evade a defender. The drum beat can be used for task simplification (see Chapter 5) slow beat that the learners are allowed to hop on, we exaggerate the need to *stick* (control) the landing in-between each hop but keep critical information the defender in the environment. It is essential that the practice environment(s) not only provides the learners with opportunities to achieve this movement solution, but also exaggerates the need for learner to search for effective solutions (see Renshaw et al., 2019), thus inviting those specific actions. Note that there have been no prescriptive instructions provided specifying precisely how learners need to complete this task.

6.4.2.3 Apply an Understanding of Co-adaptation

The successful manipulation of constraints is *nuanced*. Done successfully, this task design requires an appreciation of all the interacting elements of the system (formed by the task, environment and individual learners). The principal goal of step 3 is to ensure that the design-ing-in of constraints does not lead to *over constraining* learners and forcing them to reproduce a desired response. This is a trap that we as curriculum designers were certainly likely to have fallen into when we first started exploring these concepts of Ecological Dynamics in practice. With experience and reflection, we have found that successful manipulation of constraints requires a subtler, somewhat indirect and more patient approach. The desired actions are certainly encouraged and, indeed, solicited by the practice design. However, it is important that the actions should not be forced and should emerge as the learners search through the dynamically available (decaying and emerging) affordances within the environment. A key point is that the learners need to not only learn to identify *which* affordance to use but also *when* and then *how* to interact with them. The emergent decision to act upon an available affordance can come from exploration of the environment rather than being forced by the task constraint to interact with a specific affordance in a specific manner. When this happens, we can be more confident that functional, transferable perfor-mance solutions will emerge during learning. We have found one concept from Ecological Dynamics to be particularly useful in guiding us to successfully meet the constrain to afford principle, the notion of co-*adaptation*. Co-adaptation is the continuous interactions that emerge as learners co-adapt to each other's behaviours (i.e., other learners and individuals in the landscape). The concept of co-adaptation can also be utilised by practitioners to facilitate learners' interactions with events, objects and other properties of the performance landscape. In this way, co-adaptation can be a powerful tool to facilitate an implicit behaviour change in learners. If we continue to build on the example above, we can manipulate the *task* constraint so that pairs of learners are now required to move in tandem, connected to each other by holding a bib. The fellow teammates are the providers of an unpredictable dynamic instability that learners must co-adapt to in order to successfully achieve their intended outcomes. As the learners co-adapt against this instability, they will be perceiving information to regulate their – actions, forming synergies that are truly implicit.

In team games practice, the concept is operationalised by:

- Applying task constraints to the defending team to facilitate a behaviour change in the attacking team.
- Applying task constraints to the attacking team to facilitate a behaviour change in the defending team.
- Applying task constraints to certain team members to facilitate a behaviour change in their fellow team members.

6.4.3 Representative Learning Design

Principle 3 requires us to consider the impact that *representative learning design* (RLD) has on curriculum design. Representative design is important when specificity of learning is needed (Pinder et al., 2011). If, we are seeking to emphasise the development of physical literacy, we can employ tenets of the athletics skills model (ASM). As we note later in this book, the ASM provides us with tenets on how and when to operationalise the RLD principle and guide the development of functional movement skills and physical literacy capacities (perceptual, cognitive, emotional). As alluded to in Chapter 2, the provision of a broad variety of activities and practice landscapes is more likely to enrich learners' athletic development and promote lifelong engagement in physical activity. Paying attention to the principle of RLD ensures that learning tasks contain relevant informational constraints to elicit the emergence of functional behaviours and facilitates attunement to key affordances. The principle of RLD will be further explored in detail in future chapters, more specifically in Chapter 12 where we unpack a field hockey programme.

> **Reflection** – *When designing curriculums, we set about designing a large number and wide variety of performance landscapes for the learners to interact with. The aim was to remove the emphasis from repeating a specific game and really pushed playing a new game each week. So rather than developing expertise within one specific environment, we wanted to enhance the speed and ability of our learners to pick up and engage in a new environment, it was felt that this would have a more positive impact on the physical literacy of our learners.*

6.4.4 Repetition without Repetition (Including Variability and in(Stability))

We highlighted in Chapter 1 that children are now growing up in a risk-averse society where unstructured forms of play, interactions with nature and people's opportunities for adapting to more variable environments are constantly decreasing. The final principle challenges this tendency and promotes all practitioners to consider the concept of practice variability and requires practitioners to manage how much variability and (uncertainty and instability) they design-in their environments. Variability in practice design should promote practitioners to consider and adjust the environmental uncertainty with the aim of providing an appropriate level of (in)stability for performers. When designing practices for learning, it is essential that our changing or manipulation of constraints is to maintain system (individual, environment & task) at a critical point, *on the edge of chaos* (Bowes & Jones, 2006). This is because learners can be challenged to seek and adopt more functional behaviours in solving task problems and challenges posed by practitioners. However, it is important to be aware of the needs of each individual learner: at times, some need stability to maintain skill and consolidate learning, others may need stimulation and new challenges to take them out of their 'comfort zones'. Knowledge about 'critical values' (i.e., the amount of uncertainty that will lead to instability and the search for new solutions in learners) is important for practitioners and requires careful management and awareness of the implications for placing individuals in these critical learning regions zones. This tipping point on the edge of chaos is often the location of the optimum instability for the performer(s).

Coach Reflection – *Within our curriculums we aim to spend the significant amount of time at or just over this tipping point. It has taken a while for us as coaches (and even longer for the learner's group) to feel comfortable with experiencing this (in)stability errors within our practice environment and reframing them if not as a positive sign, or at the very least an opportunity to learn. Providing games with a wide access point, or as we would term it, a low floor and a high ceiling, allowing the learners to engage at their level of (in)stability had a positive effect on participant engagement. In fact, we have observed learners being implicitly drawn to a level of (in)stability that they can positively engaged with.*

Physical literacy provides an important foundation for learners faced with new challenges and problems to solve in play, sport and physical activity (Rudd et al., 2020; O'Sullivan et al., 2020). There are occasions where it may be advantageous to design-in a low amount of informational uncertainty in a task. For example, we may wish to design practice tasks that do not promote any additional pattern forming or system re-organisation. Task stabilisation provides environments that allow learners to tune in to the information in a performance environment or to consolidate what they already know about the performance environment. In contrast, there will always be a 'critical value' above which the environment will contain too much uncertainty, and as a result it will become inherently chaotic and unmanageable (Davids et al., 2003). It is important for practitioners to be cautious when designing in this much uncertainty: in effect to focus on the periodisation of the skill learning process. The periodisation of skill training has received some recent interest (Otte, Miller & Klatt, 2019) and is a concept we will certainly be exploring further as we attempt to become more systematic and deliberate when designing-in variability to our curriculum.

6.5 Concluding Remarks

In this chapter we drew attention to the challenging role of designing learning environments in play, physical activity and sport programmes to support the ongoing development of physical literacy. We conclude the chapter by drawing the reader's attention to two considerations that may be particularly useful during the design of such learning environments. The first liberating breakthrough is to appreciate the *trade-offs* associated with learning design decisions made. The process of learning design is a complex and messy endeavour, and often there is no perfect solution. As we have suggested previously, there is no *magic bullet w*hen it comes to understanding how best to manipulate task constraints to enrich learning (Renshaw et al., 2019). We will explore examples of these necessary trade-offs in more detail within the case study chapters later in the book. The second element to consider is the realisation that, despite rigorous planning, we can still only make educated predictions of how the different elements of the learning system (formed by the individual, task and environment) will interact. The non-linear, emergent nature of complex biological systems makes learners' interactions with the affordances of a learning landscape difficult to predict. This property of learners should alleviate the pressure that practitioners may place on themselves to provide perfect (ideal) learning environments from the outset. It does however establish the need for practitioners to be agile and adaptable, and highly attuned to the immediate needs of learners for enriching their physical literacy, in order to adjust task designs appropriately, based on the learner-environment interactions observed in the moment.

References

Araújo, D. & Davids, K. (2011). What exactly is acquired during skill acquisition? *Journal of Consciousness Studies, 18,* 7–23.

Bernstein, A. (1967). *The coordination and regulation of movements.* London: Pergamon Press.

Bowes, I. & Jones, R. L. (2006). Working at the edge of chaos: Understanding coaching as a complex, interpersonal system. *The Sport Psychologist, 20*(2), 235–245.

Chow, J.-Y., Davids, K., Button, C. & Renshaw, I. (2016). *Nonlinear pedagogy in skill acquisition: An introduction.* London: Routledge.

Davids, K., Glazier, P., Araujo, D. & Bartlett, R. (2003). Movement systems as dynamical systems: The functional role of variability and its implications for sports medicine. *Sports Medicine, 33*(4), 245–260.

Greenwood, D., Davids, K. & Renshaw, I. (2014). Experiential knowledge of expert coaches can help identify informational constraints on performance of dynamic interceptive actions. *Journal of Sports Sciences, 32*(4), 328–335.

Newcombe, D., Roberts, W., Renshaw, I. & Davids, K. (2019). The effectiveness of constraints-led training on skill development in interceptive sports: A systematic review (Clark, McEwan and Christie) - a commentary. *International Journal of Sports Science and Coaching, 14*(2), 241–254.

Otte, F. W., Miller, S. & Klatt, S. (2019). skill training periodization in "Specialist" sports coaching—An introduction of the "PoST" framework for skill development. *Frontiers in Sport and Active Living, 1,* 61.

O'Sullivan, M., Davids, K., Woods, C. T., Rothwell, M. & Rudd, J. (2020). Conceptualizing physical literacy within an ecological dynamics framework. *Quest, 72*(4), 1–15.

Pinder, R., Davids, K., Renshaw, I. & Araújo, D. (2011). Representative learning design and functionality of research and practice in sport. *Journal of Sport and Exercise Psychology, 33,* 146–155.

Renshaw, I., Davids, K., Newcombe, D. & Roberts, W. (2019). *The constraints led approach: Principles for sports coaching and practice design.* London: Routledge.

Rudd, J. R., Pesce, C., Strafford, B. W. & Davids, K. (2020). Physical literacy-a journey of individual enrichment: An ecological dynamics rationale for enhancing performance and physical activity in all. *Frontiers in Psychology, 11*, 1904.

Woods, C., Rothwell, M., Rudd, J., Robertson, S. & Davids, K. (2020). Representative co-design: Utilising a source of experiential knowledge for athlete development and performance preparation. *Psychology of Sport & Exercise, 52*, 101804.

Woods, C. T., Rudd, J., Robertson, S., Davids, K. (2020). Wayfinding: How ecological perspectives of navigating dynamic environments can enrich our understanding of the learner and the learning process in sport. *Sports Medicine – Open, 6*, 51.

7

THE ATHLETIC SKILLS MODEL

Enhancing Physical Literacy across the Lifespan

Geert Savelsbergh and René Wormhoudt

7.1 Introduction

As highlighted in Chapter 1 today's generation of children is significantly less fit than, and do not move as well as, their peers from 40 years ago (Vandorpe et al., 2011) due to lifestyles that can inhibit meaningful activity. A longitudinal study with children aged between 5 and 7 years showed that those with low movement ability are more likely to be less fit 5 years later, compared to children who are competent movers (Hands, 2008). The development of movement skills may never have been so important to children's all-round health and well-being. It is most important that foundational movements and all aspects of physical literacy be optimally developed through participation in enriched environments. How can practitioners 'enrich' a physical education, sport or physical activity programme to enhance physical literacy? Through highlights in this book so far one might be tempted to think on a grand scale of continually upgrading activity environments such as venues, playing surfaces, alongside adopting a coach/teacher development programme to transition to the adoption of a Nonlinear Pedagogy (NLP). The first of these may not be feasible due to finances and lack of space and available facilities. Our second idea focuses on the need for contemporary pedagogical frameworks to be developed, based on understanding of current social and cultural changes in society. The development of contemporary pedagogies is advocated, but this takes time and should be a continual cycle of reflection, discussion and action. Following on from our introduction of constraint-led approach (CLA), NLP and Environmental Design Principles (EDP), we introduce an alternative to traditional programme structures, the Athletics Skills Model (ASM), which emanated from observations of developmental sporting histories of elite athletes in professional sports[1]. The ASM proposes how a diverse range of sport experiences can enrich later specialisation in a targeted sport (Wormhoudt et al., 2018).

The ASM goal is to provide a suitable framework to structure developmental movement programmes fostering physical literacy. The programme long-term goal is to educate and develop each individual's capabilities to seek out and engage in lifelong physical activity and sport participation by maintaining a balance between performance, fitness, and health across the lifespan. The ASM framework as advocates the need for practitioners to consider learners' non-linear developmental trajectories. In order to reach this goal, the ASM's pedagogical principles of complement a NLP. Practitioners using the ASM employ and have a deep appreciation for: (1) concentric teaching methods, (2) exploiting possibilities of transfer between participation in different sports and activities, and (3) creating challenging in- and outdoor environments for learner. Each of these tools, separately, or in combination with each other, will increase learners' exploration of the environment. Through this process ASM experiences will create opportunities for more functional variations and adaptation of movement skills. Before we move on to show how the ASM and the NLP approaches can be combined, the ASM is explained, followed by an overview of recent developments with respect to contemporary motor learning theory.

7.2 The Athletic Skills Model for Fostering and Enhancing Movement Experiences

The ASM is based on the approach that body and mind are unified, and best appreciated as a complex, adaptive system (Wormhoudt, Teunissen & Savelsbergh, 2012; Savelsbergh & Wormhoudt, 2019). The basics of this model are informed by the combination of theoretical ideas from Ecological Dynamics, key scientific findings, and experiential knowledge from extensive practice in (high-performance) sport (Wormhoudt et al., 2018). The ASM programme introduces the following development framework:

- First, the child needs to become a versatile 'good mover', with movement being associated with fun, pleasure, and enjoyment (a)[2]; subsequently, she/he may wish to develop into an athlete (b); as an athlete the child will specialise in one sport (c), and could finally develop into an absolute specialist within this sport (d). So, the key of the ASM is: first become an athlete, only then specialise as an athlete.

This sequence is not fixed by age, but more or less to functional skills required for achieving these future aims, which could include becoming an elite or recreational athlete. The ASM programme seeks to create a stable basis for performance by developing a physical literacy on which a healthy physical active lifestyle and/or sporting career can be founded and developed. The model builds on the other established models such as the talent model of Bloom (1985), the sport diversification ideas of Côté (1999), Côté et al. (2011) and Côté and Erickson (2015), the different pedagogical aims of Balyi and Hamilton (2004), and the early engagement idea of Ford et al. (2009) (see Table 2.4, p. 46 in Wormhoudt et al., 2018). The ASM strives to support the development of fitter, adaptable, more rounded individuals who will establish a longer (professionally or recreationally) active lifestyle. As a consequence of more variation in movement learning experiences, in comparison to monotonic traditional programmes, the chances of getting injured are decreased significantly (practical methods are explained in Section 7.5 of this chapter). As a result, individuals have more performance-related growth opportunities, which can enhance their personal development and general health and well-being. These aims fit very nicely into the description of physical literacy, especially the first stage – to become a good mover (first an athlete) – which should enhance the physical literacy from an early age onwards. The child is not 'forced' into an early specialisation trajectory but acquires a broad range of functional movement skills through movement education and free play, for instance, by experiencing a diversity of play activities and sports[3]. This is known as the

ASM continuum. It's an adaptive, Multi- and Donorsport programme that can then be related to any specific sport programme (see Section 7.5 and for elaborative description and explanation of ASM Continuum see Chapter 6 in Wormhoudt et al., 2018).

7.3 Motor Learning

As we covered in Chapter 4 over the last two decades wealth of motor learning research has been conducted but not integrated into talent development models with an aim to increase the physical literacy of people (Wormhoudt et al., 2018: Chapter 4). Traditionally, the motor learning process has been modelled sequentially. In early learning phases, one learns about the movement execution through verbal instructions from a parent or teacher, performing only some parts of a movement, which costs a lot of attentional effort. In the next phase, there is more refinement and improved control, which needs less conscious control, whilst movement execution requires less effort. In the third phase, automaticity of movement control is putatively achieved, providing room to perform other tasks in addition to, and at the same time as, the main movement. This type of traditional approach to the motor learning process, however, requires a qualified supervisor, teacher, or coach to prescribe a putative 'ideal' movement pattern and reduce any deviations from these technical templates. This model of learning is still dominant in the daily practical teaching of motor skills in physical education and sports programmes. However, as we noted earlier, in the last 25 years attention to contemporary theories of motor learning and development (e.g. Ecological Dynamics; Newell CLA, 1986; Smith and Thelen's (1995) work on dynamic systems theory, e.g. 1995) have initiated a new focus on learning designs (See Chapters 4 and 5). These alternative forms of learning do not necessarily need the presence of a qualified supervisor, but can be realised by creating environments that 'guide' and 'challenge' the child or athlete in such a way that desirable movement outcomes will be achieved. Underpinning the design of these environments is the aim to support learning as a process of discovering, exploring, and improving motor skills. Essential in this learning approach is the concept of functional variability (Savelsbergh et al., 2006), a key element of NLP on which we discuss in the next section.

7.4 Principles of Nonlinear Pedagogy

As discussed in Chapter 4, coaches and physical education teachers are designers of learning environment. That is in order to enhance the performance, the practice must be designed in such a way that it allows the performer (e.g. athlete, or child or elderly) to exploit learning environments that promote adaptive performance behaviours (Correia et al., 2018). A central key element of NLP (Chapter 5) is to manipulate constraints in such a way that learning is facilitated (Chow et al., 2006; Renshaw et al., 2016). The learning designs created by constraints manipulation should facilitate exploration of functional possible movement solutions. These possible solutions increase adaptability. This way, the process of self-organisation and the less conscious control of movement (more implicit learning) is promoted, leading to individualised functional solutions (Correia et al., 2018).

In the NLP, the stages of motor learning as suggested by Bernstein (1967) coordination, control, and skill are honoured. That is a freezing, freeing, and exploiting of the degrees of freedom is encouraged by the design of a learning environment. A design can enhance the skill adaptation of the performer through self-regulation (self-organisation) in search for more functional performance solutions (Araújo & Davids, 2011). This movement variability is crucial because it offers different solutions for learners to explore. Another important consequence of NLP is that it helps the learner by exploring the redundancy of the movement system and the possibilities for transfer of movement. The positive transfer of movements is a key aspect of ASM to which we return in the next section, discussing how principles of NLP are relevant for the ASM methods in application.

7.5 How Does ASM Enhance Physical Literacy?

To foster physical literacy, we should create learning environments that provide room for exploration, allows emergences of (functional) variability, and foster movement adaptability in beginners and advanced learners. In the process of solving motor problems the performer can find movement solutions that lead to new and highly functional, creative behaviours (Orth et al., 2017). By encouraging greater diversification of capabilities in a population of learners, the greater the adaptability and creativity of the developmental system will be, overall. These ideas are aligned with the principles of NLP briefly outline in Chapter 5.

The ASM advocates three major avenues to enrich movement experiences to foster physical literacy, namely:

1. make use of the concentric approach to movement skills acquisition;
2. exploit the transferability of movements;
3. create challenging environments from a constraints-led perspective.

In all three aims, the NLP principles can be used for guidance to allow the emergence of more effective functional movement solutions that aim to structure learning tasks and environments that allow the individual to solve their own movement problems. The freely emerging co-adaptation amongst individuals involved in the learning system enhances creativity and adaptability of the learners, and as a consequence, develops physical literacy in quantity and in quality

7.6 The Concentric Approach

What does a concentric development mean in the process of acquiring basic movement skills? It means that, for example, one basic movement skill like hitting a ball in tennis, can be developed by practising and experiencing all types of hitting as applied in other sports and activities. For instance, a versatile concentric approach to hitting in tennis is: hitting a baseball, playing table tennis, playing golf, Lacrosse, or performing a volleyball smash (Wormhoudt et al., 2018). In the ASM the basic movement skill of 'hitting' an object is strongly correlated with performance of related skills like: throwing, catching, and aiming. These related skills are all combined in one of the 10 basic movement skills. So, a concentric approach for hitting also means learning to throw, to catch and aim an object in a diversified way

In contrast, in the traditional linear approach to motor learning, the next step is pre-set (based on some putative technical model) and is ultimately designed for only one purpose, to achieve a goal or execute an exercise, for example, producing a single outcome, from rolling (rotating the body) to a somersault. Such a linear development programme is inherently limiting and mainly designed for the execution of a specific exercise. In contrast a concentric programme is designed for the intensification and development of functional human abilities or skills, which will amplify meaningful movement experiences in a variety of contexts. This way an increase in a learner's information-movement couplings are encouraged leading ultimate to access new movement possibilities (Wormhoudt et al., 2018; Savelsbergh & Wormhoudt, 2019). Because the athlete can readily realise a diversity of actions across a range of contexts, learning in the concentric phase of the ASM can also support a higher degree of skill adaptability, leading to unique and functional solutions (i.e. creativity) emerging during game play (Santos et al., 2016) (See Chapter 14). For instance, rolling (rotating) is possible in three planes around multiple axes, such as when performing a pirouette in ballet, pivots in games like basketball, a judo throw, cartwheels, taekwondo spinning kicks, and a somersault in gymnastics. The concentric approach encourages diversity within functional movement skills but also offers an entrance to transferabilities.

7.7 The Exploitation of Transfer Processes

The ASM principles are predicated on results of previous research, which have shown that transfer processes directly increase both the degree of primary task learning and inter-task similarity; this has been attributed to both response generalisation and learning-how-to-learn. Findings showed the capability of an individual of performing a task successfully and his/her ability to transfer this performance to another task in learning. This key idea supports the idea that learning one task extensively can be supported by learning another task that contains similar elements and can causes improvement in the premier task. As stated earlier, the ability to adaptively and flexibly modify movement behaviour is a key objective contributing to the varied repertoire of skilled actions. In order to achieve this objective, ASM exploits this transferability of movements and for that purpose brings in the concepts of Multisports and Donorsports.

Multisports experiences are often linked to the concept of sampling of Côté, Lidor and Hackfort (2009). It is already well known and suggested that practising different sports is beneficial for health and social reasons but, also for developing better performance in a target sport. This diversity of experience may lead to numerous positive growth and developmental opportunities (Côté et al., 2009). This key idea has clear evidence to support it, as we discussed earlier in this section (Barth et al., 2020), whether from an unstructured or coach-led perspective. However, this idea of sport sampling is not 100% identical with the ASM concept of Multisport and has been refined.

Within the ASM approach, Multisports is redefined as playing and sampling many other sports of which the basic movement skills of these sport are *not or almost not present* in a target (main or selected) sport. That way the amount of functional movement skills experienced and learned is extended and improved. As a consequence, this more varied and extensive Multisports experience enhances the level of physical literacy in a learner.

The concept of Donorsports refers to sports or activities that are selected to contribute to performance in the 'chosen' target sport that consists of the same functional movement skills. This means that practising a Donorsport will contribute to elements of the target sport and thus your expertise level in that particular sport (see for elaborate discussion Wormhoudt et al., 2018). Strafford et al. (2018) argued that Donorsports and target sports may share parts of the same affordance landscape (thereby inviting similar movement patterns from learners). So Multi- and Donorsports can be seen as complementary in order to cover *all* functional movement skills and, as such, forms a strong foundation for physical literacy. Recent research supports the Donorsport idea and shows a positive transfer for climbing from one environment to another one (Seifert et al., 2016) and from futsal to football (Oppici et al., 2018).

In the first example, the capability of climbers who had trained in indoor climbing to climb on outdoor icefalls for the first time was examined. Participants climbing fluency (performance) and number of exploratory actions (where the individual touches a hold with a hand or ice-axe only to withdraw it to find another or the same anchorage) were compared. It was found that the novice ice-climbers could successfully complete the ice route – supported by a general transfer of skill between indoor and ice climbing. Whilst the emotional and psychological requirements for climbing icefalls would have been significantly different from those required to climb indoor walls, many of the underlying movement skills were similar (Seifert et al., 2016). In this case, evidence suggests that indoor climbing as a Donorsport can help prepare individuals for safer exploration and more effective participation in ice climbing.

In a second example, it was investigated how learning a passing skill with futsal or association football task constraints influenced transfer to a new task. Fourteen-year-old players with either a background in futsal (the futsal group) or football (the football group) each performed two tasks. One task involved playing a small-sided game that is playing in a small area with the futsal ball. The second task was a football-like task (large playing area with the football). Players' passing accuracy and their orientation of attention were assessed during the two tasks. The futsal group improved their passing accuracy from the futsal-like to the football-like task, and they were more accurate than football players. For the football group, passing accuracy remained stable across the two tasks and it was similar to the futsal group in the futsal-like task. These findings showed a transfer (and adaptability) from performing passes in a small playing area with a short time to act – futsal task constraints – to a larger playing area with a longer time – football task constraints – than vice versa. In other words, futsal can be considered as a Donorsport for football.

The concentric approach can be applied in Multisports as well as in the Donorsports, which provides the child, athlete, elderly, instructors with a very wide range of options for learning designs. These options are used by ASM practitioners to make tailored structural programmes (see for elaborative descriptions, Wormhoudt et al., 2018). This type of designed environment can 'help' to apply concentric approach and to encourage and exploit transfers possibilities.

7.8 Creating Challenging Environments

The environment in which learning and (creative) activities take place, should provide the child or athlete the ground on which creativity can more *readily flourish* (Hasirci & Demirkan, 2003: Runco, 2004). How can these motor activities, be promoted? In order to achieve this aim of 'readily flourishing', the ASM design can be used to build a completely new environment: PLAYCE and The Skills Garden. PLAYCE and the Skills Garden can be described as attractive, innovative, and sustainable outdoor facilities that can be used for leisure, playing, education, training, practice, and rehabilitation. All elements are modular and can be implemented on existing or new locations. This public facility, conforming to the ASM principles, enables an all-round motoric development by the use of all 10 Basic Movement Skills as defined by Wormhoudt et al. (2018), such as balancing, climbing, throwing, catching, and jumping. This concept of PLAYCE and Skill Garden finds its foundation in the theoretical model of Newell (1986) and provides the opportunities to apply the NLP approach in order to enhance learners' physical literacy. The Skill Garden provides many different environmental constraints and as such provides several opportunities for movement exploration, through manipulation of movement scaling opportunities. It is well known in scientific research that scaling can be used to influence the learning process. For instance, in a study of Timmermans and collaborators the influence of scaling court-size and net height on children's tennis performance was examined (Timmermans et al., 2015). Ten-year-old boys performed a 30-minute match in four different conditions, where court-size and/or net height was scaled using a ratio based on the differences in temporal demands between the children and the adult game. The players hit *more* winners; *more* forced errors, played *more* volleys, struck *more* shots from a comfortable height and played in a *more* forward court position when the net is scaled. Scaling both the court and net led to a faster children's game, more closely approximating what is typical of the adult game. Importantly, children enjoyed playing on the standard court–scaled net condition more than standard adult conditions.

In a second tennis example, a simple manipulation of scaling factor, that lowering the net height to 0.65 m and 0.52 m led to players *adopting without prior instruction* a more attacking style of play, which is support for the Nonlinear pedagogical approach. A significant increase in the number of winners was observed, without a commensurate increase in errors and more shots struck inside the baseline. Lower nets also led to a greater percentage of successful first serves (Limpens et al., 2018).

The concept of Skill Garden has been installed at the professional Football club AFC Ajax, Football Medical Centre at Zeist and at the KNVB, Dutch National Football Association Campus in the Netherlands (an outdoor and indoor facility). The Skills Garden stimulates challenges and provides a pleasurable movement experience that stimulates adaptability (see for elaborative description Chapter 10 of Wormhoudt et al., 2018). It focuses on health, fitness, and sports and activities and can be used for leisure, playing, education, training, practice, and rehabilitation, and therefore contributes to the enhancement of the physical literacy by making use of the CLA and NLP principles.

7.9 Roads to Physical Literacy from an ASM Point of View

In order to foster physical literacy, we should be able to create learning environments that foster adaptability. In the process of solving motor problems the performer can find movement solutions that lead to new and highly functional (creative) behaviour (Orth et al., 2017). By encouraging greater diversification of capabilities in a population of learners, the greater the adaptability and creativity of the developmental system overall. Considering those points, the ASM advocates three major roads to achieve higher levels of the physical literacy: by using the concentric approach to movement skills acquisition, by exploiting the transferability of movements, and by creating challenging environments.

Applying these three 'ASM roads', each separately or in combination will increase the level of physical literacy as well as creativity and adaptability. For instance, for a child, the concentric approach and Multisport can expand her/his potential for future development of performance into adulthood. For the recreational mover, the concentric approach can be applied by experiencing Multisports, or a concentric approach to skill learning (e.g. balancing) in the Skills Garden. For elite athletes, Donorsports, carried out for instance in a Skills Garden, will increase the level of expertise as a result of acquiring a wider network of perceptual-motor skills that 'supports' the possibility of emergence of a greater diversity of movement solutions and problems they can be adapted to (Gullich, 2017). Finally, the current chapter advocated that the ASM serves as a suitable model to structure (developmental) movement programmes to enhance physical literacy with a view of supporting lifelong physical activity participation and seeks to maintain a balance between performance, fitness, and health.

Notes

1 A longitudinal study in the United States (Olympian Report, 1984–1998, Hill et al., 2002) concluded, amongst other things, that Olympic medallists practised on average 3.4 sports per person at school and 3.1 sports outside school. This could mean that there is a relation between practising several different sports (e.g. acquiring many different basic movement skills) and reaching the top in the target sport.
2 We developed a movement track that can measure the movement abilities of children and can be used in order to establish the level of fundamental movement abilities (Hoeboer et al., 2016; 2018).
3 Several researchers highlighted the relationship between good movement skills and sport participation (e.g. Barnett et al., 2016; Logan et al., 2015).

References

Araújo, D. & Davids, K. (2011). What exactly is acquired during skill acquisition? *Journal of Consciousness Studies, 18*, 7–23.

Balyi, I. & Hamilton, A. (2004). *Long-term athlete development: Trainability in childhood and adolescence. windows of opportunity. optimal trainability.* Victoria: National Coaching Institute British Columbia & Advanced Training and Performance Ltd., Victoria.

Barnett, L. M., Stodden, D., Cohen, K. E., Smith, J. J. et al. (2016) Fundamental movement skills: An important focus. *Journal of Teaching in Physical Education, 35*, 219–225.

Barth, M., Güllich, A., Raschner, C. & Emrich, E. (2020). The path to international medals: A supervised machine learning approach to explore the impact of coach-led sport-specific and non-specific practice. *PloS One, 15*(9).

Bernstein, N.A. (1967). The co-ordination and regulation of movements. Pergamon Press, Oxford.

Bloom, B. S. (1985). *Developing talent in Young people.* New York: Ballantine Books.

Chow, J.Y., Davids, K., Button, C., Shuttleworth, R., Renshaw, I. & Araújo, D. (2006). Nonlinear pedagogy: A constraints-led framework to understand emergence of game play and skills. nonlinear dynamics. *Psychology and Life Sciences, 10*(1), 71–104.

Correia, V., Carvalho, J., Araújo, D., Pereira, E. & Davids, K. (2018). Principles of nonlinear pedagogy in sport practice. *Physical Education and Sport Pedagogy, 24*, 117–132. doi:10.1080/17408989.2018.1552673.

Côté, J. (1999). The influence of the family in the development of talent in sport. *The Sport Psychologist, 13*, 395–417.

Côté, J. & Erickson, K. (2015). Diversification and deliberate play during the sampling years. In J. Baker & D. Farrow(Eds.). *Routledge handbook of sport expertise* (pp. 305–316). London: Routledge.

Côté, J., Lidor, R. & Hackfort, D. (2009). ISSP position stand: To sample or to specialize? Seven postulates about youth sport activities that lead to continued participation and elite performance. *International Journal of Sport and Exercise Psychology, 7*(1), 7–17.

Ford, P. R., Ward, P., Hodges, N. J. & Williams, M. A. (2009). The role of deliberate practice and play in career progression in sport: The early engagement hypothesis. *High Ability Studies, 20*(1), 65–75.

Gullich, A. (2017). International medallists and non-medallists developmental sport: A match pairs analysis. *Journal of Sport Sciences, 35*, 2281–2288.

Hands, B. (2008). Changes in motor skill and fitness measures among children with high and low motor competence: A five-year longitudinal study. *Journal of Science and Medicine in Sport, 11*(2), 155–162. doi:10.1016/j.jsams.2007.02.012.

Hasirci, D. & Demirkan, H. (2003). Creativity in learning environments: The case of two sixth grade art rooms. *Journal of Creative Behavior, 37*, 17–41.

Hill, R., McConnell, A., Forster, T. & Moore, J. (2002). *The path to excellence: A comprehensive view of development of U.S. Olympians who competed from 1984 to 1998*. USOC, Performance Services Department.

Hoeboer, J., DeVries, S., Krijger-Hombergen, M., Wormdhoudt, R., Drent, A., Krabben, K. & Savelsbergh, G. J. P. (2016). Validity of an athletic skills track among 6- to 12-year old children. *Journal of Sport Sciences, 34*, 2095–2105.

Hoeboer, J. J. A. A. M., Ongena, G., Krijger-Hombergen, M., Stolk, E., Savelsbergh, G. J. P. & De Vries, S. I. (2018). The athletic skills track: Age- and gender-related normative values of a motor skills test for 4- to 12-year-old children. *Journal of Science and Medicine in Sport, 21*, 975–979. doi:10.1016/j.jsams.2018.01.014.

Limpens, V., Buszard, T., Shoemaker, E., Savelsbergh, G. J. & Reid, M. (2018). Scaling constraints in junior tennis: The influence of net height on skilled players' match-play performance. *Research Quarterly for Exercise and Sport, 89*(1), 1–10.

Logan, S. W., Webster, E. K., Getchell, N., Pfeiffer, K. & Robinson, L. E. (2015). Relationship between fundamental motor skill competence and physical activity during childhood and adolescence: A systematic review. *Kinesiology Review, 4*, 416–426.

Newell, K. (1986). Constraints on the development of coordination. In: M. Wade & H. T. Whiting (Eds.), *Motor development in children: Aspects of coordination and control*. Dordrecht, Netherlands: Martinus Nijhoff.

Oppici, L., Panchuk, D., Serpiello, F. R. & Farrow, D. (2018). Futsal task constraints promote transfer of passing skill to soccer task constraints. *European Journal of Sport Science, 18*(7), 947–954.

Orth, D., van der Kamp, J., Memmert, D. & Savelsbergh, G. (2017). Creative motor actions as emerging from movement variability. *Frontiers in Psychology, 8*(1903).

Renshaw, I., Araújo, D., Button, C., Chow, J. Y., Davids, K. & Moy, B. (2016). Why the constraints-led approach is not teaching games for understanding: A clarification. *Physical Education and Sport Pedagogy, 21*(5), 459–480.

Runco, M. A. (2004). Creativity. *Annual Review Psychology, 55*, 657–87.

Santos, S. D., Memmert, D., Sampaio, J. & Leite, N. (2016). The spawns of creative behavior in team sports: A creativity developmental framework. *Frontiers in Psychology, 7*, 1282.

Savelsbergh, G. J. P., Vander Kamp, J. & Rosengren, K. S. (2006). Functional variability in perceptual-movement development. In K. Davids, S. Bennett & K. Newell (Eds.) *Variability in the movement systems: A multi-disciplinary perspective*. Urbana Champaign, IL: Human Kinetics.

Savelsbergh, G. J. P. & Wormhoudt, R. (2019). Creating adaptive athletes: The athletic skills model for enhancing physical literacy as a foundation for expertise. *Movement & Sport Science, 102*, 31–38.

Seifert, L., Wattebled, L., Orth, D., L'Hermette, M., Boulanger, J. & Davids, K. (2016). Skill transfer specificity shapes perception and action under varying environmental constraints. *Human Movement Science, 48*, 132–141.

Strafford, B. W., Van Der Steen, P., Davids, K., & Stone, J. A. (2018). Parkour as a donor sport for athletic development in youth team sports: insights through an ecological dynamics lens. *Sports medicine-open, 4*(1), 1-6.

Thelen, E. & Smyth, L. B. (1995). *A dynamic systems approach to development of cognition and action*. Bradford, PA: Bradford Books.

Timmermans, E., De Water, J., Kachel, K., Reid, M., Farrow, D. & Savelsbergh, G. J. P. (2015). The effect of equipment scaling on children's sport performance: The case for tennis. *Journal of Sport Sciences, 33*, 1093–1100.

Vandorpe, B., Vandendriessche, J., Lefevre, J., Pion, J., Vaeyens, R., Matthys, S., Philippaerts, R. & Lenoir, M. (2011). The KörperkoordinationsTest für Kinder: Reference values and suitability for 6–12-year-old children in Flanders. *Scandinavian Journal of Medicine and Science in Sports, 21*, 378–388.

Wormhoudt, R., Savelsbergh, G. J. P., Teunissen, J. W. & Davids, K. W. (2018). *The athletic skills model for optimizing talent development through movement education*. London: Routledge.

Wormhoudt, R., Teunissen, J. W. & Savelsbergh, G. J. P. (2012). *Het Athletic Skills Model voor een optimale talent ontwikkeling*. (Athletic skills model for optimizing talent development). Arko Sports Media.

SECTION III

Further Considerations and Future Direction of Research and Practice in Physical Literacy

Section 3: Introduction

Over the last two decades, 'testing' has become a central focus as a way of making teachers 'more accountable' and underpins a political desire to 'improve standards'. However, testing has had a negative effect on educational landscapes with teachers, students and parents suffering the consequence and its effect as embodied and emotional experiences. Just like the race to the bottom in junior sport, testing from the age of five in many (but not all) Western schools that compares students to a norm, has led to negative reactions from these teachers, parents and perhaps most importantly, children (Lingard, Thompson & Sellar, 2016). It is therefore hard to reconcile the desire to improve the experiences of children with the significant stress and anxiety they cause to all stakeholders. An additional problem, is that in line with the insights of Kaplan (1991) as discussed in Chapter 1, being a child today is a very different experience to that of their grandparents as they are subjected to greater academic work at earlier ages. The pressure put on children by parents and teachers means they have less opportunity to play and less opportunity to direct their own play to develop physical literacy. A knock-on effect of a default assessment of teaching quality by proxy is that often teachers feel compelled to teach to the test with a reduction in the promotion of autonomous learning opportunities as they become more and more controlling. This has a significant impact on motivational orientation, and it is well established in educational psychology, that when the controlling aspect of an external event (such as formal testing) is more relevant to the recipient than the information it provides, that, that event will tend to decrease in motivation.

Current trends in testing have unfortunately permeated the physical education landscape as schools are routinely blamed for (a) any failures of the national team in the current international tournament; (b) the poor health of the nation and (c) low levels of physical activity of 'children today' who spend significant time each day playing computer and video games. As in teaching in the classroom, teaching through the physical education has endured calls for more 'testing' to drive up 'performance', whether that be movement skills, school sport teams win ratio or the physical activity levels of children.

In Chapter 8, we highlight how tests of physical literacy have been attempted based on reductionist methods, where the discrete 'components' of physical literacy are measured using checklists rather than through assessment based on the process. Essentially, physical literacy has been substituted using terms like fundamental movement skills, which are purported to be the building blocks upon which more complex movements and skills can be built. Such an approach appears to be in-line with the milestone or maturational perspective in favour in the 1930s where development was viewed where development was viewed as an 'orderly and sequenced development process driven by a biological or genetic clock (Haywood & Getchell, 2019). Underpinning this idea is that we can assess an individual's physical literacy using standards tests and against an age-based set of norms favoured in the last century (Haywood & Getchell, 2019). It seems we have gone back to the future to test children's movement capabilities. However, such a linear approach to developing physical literacy is questioned by more contemporary views in motor development, where the interaction between each individual and the environments in which learning occurs the context of development (Adolph, Hoch & Cole, 2018) is viewed as crucial to developmental pathways and emergent skilled repertoires. Adopting such an approach means that practitioners and researchers acknowledge that 'skills stutter into infants' repertoires, with variable trajectories that oscillate between skill expression and non-expression over several days, weeks, or months' (Adolph et al., 2018, p. 702). In the chapter, we therefore question this reductionist approach and pose some key questions and provide some potential answers for practitioners and researchers to consider when measuring and subsequently designing interventions to support the development of an individual's physical literacy.

In the final chapter of this section, we summarise what we have learned so far and provide some pointers as to the way forward for practitioners and researchers interested in physical literacy. Drawing upon historical socio-cultural constraints we argue that practitioners and educators have a duty to support children on their physical literacy journey and that this aim has to move beyond current pedagogical practices that turn children off from being physically active. We argue that an essential requirement underpinning any relevant approach that could be adopted by practitioners needs to be based on physical literacy as a journey that has enriched environments that encourage exploration and autonomy as its central pillars. To that end we conclude with some recommendations to support the emergence of functional, not fundamental movement skills through active engagement with the world, supporting increasingly skilful interactions with the environment.

8

A MORE HOLISTIC WAY OF MEASURING PHYSICAL LITERACY

James Rudd, Will Roberts, and Daniel Newcombe

8.1 A Thought on Measurement to Support Physical Literacy

In previous chapters, we have argued that socio-cultural and environmental constraints such as the advent of technological advances and changes in working patterns have resulted in reduced levels of physical activity, and a paucity of movement skills in much of the developed world. This has significant potential social and economic costs for society and is driving a worldwide focus on young people's physical literacy. Historically, physical literacy has developed naturally through play but we are now living in a world where we see play deprivation.

In our quest to develop individual physical literacy over the last decade (Canada, Australia, the United Kingdom amongst others) we have had a tendency to want outcomes that we can measure in order that we might 'prove' that policy, funding, physical activity intervention or teaching and coaching have had a positive impact. This is particularly prevalent in highly structured and professionalised sports training programmes and in educational contexts where pressure is applied to redress many of the issues of physical inactivity we have presented in this book. However, when we reflect upon an Ecological Dynamics conceptualisation of physical literacy as set out in Chapter 2, then the question of whether we should, or indeed can, measure physical literacy emerges as a focal point. Perhaps, it is not a question of whether we should measure physical literacy, but rather that we, as practitioners and researchers, should consider an alternative understanding of what counts as measurement. As postulated in this book, let us accept that physical literacy reflects an individual, and holistic notion of one's disposition to choose how to respond to an environment, or context, based on our capabilities to do so, and then perhaps it is not too far a stretch of the imagination to suggest that the interaction with the environment, is in fact a measure of an individual's physical literacy.

Consider this example:

*If two people are presented with stepping stones to cross a fast-flowing river, the affordance of crossability is always present. However, in this example, the possibility to act on that affordance is only an option for **Person A**. This is partly due to the properties of the environment such as the distance between the stones and the characteristics of the surface of the stone such as its size, shape, slippiness (due to moss and how wet it is) but it is also complemented by the effectivities of **Person A**. **Person B** has different effectivities to **Person A** and these do not provide a goodness of fit between the environment and the task (to cross the river). As a result Person **B** will have to find another way to cross the river or will have to be supported in crossing.*

The question we must consider is if **Person A** is able to do something, that **Person B** does not do, does that make **Person A** more physically literate than **Person B**? This is a contention in the academic literature, for many the answer is yes and that we should intervene to support **Person B** and develop their capacities through intervention. In time, it is argued that unless there are structural limitations, such as height, weight, etc., **Person B** will develop effectivities to actualise the affordance to enable them to cross the river. In terms of measurement, there are several challenges here that need careful consideration. First, physical literacy measurement tools are not currently affordance based and therefore there are validity issues as these may not be measuring the children's true movement potential. Secondly, when measuring physical literacy how can we avoid reverting to the very thing that Margaret Whitehead said she wanted to move away from, that is, performance-driven curricula and sports programmes. In this chapter our aim is to explore these challenges, first, to see whether it might be possible to create a valid and reliable affordance-based measure of physical literacy and secondly, to see whether we can use this to inform the development of interventions that do not lead to performative-based curricula.

8.2 Physical Literacy Measurement around the World

If used appropriately, measurement is a powerful tool that can provide the practitioner with important data about how to support the development of the learner. Measurement in physical literacy is used all over the world to capture children's physical literacy; in Canada the measurement of physical literacy has focused on quantification of separate physical, affective and cognitive domains (Way et al., 2014, p. 23), whilst in countries which propose that physical literacy is the integration of physical, psychological, social, and cognitive skill, its measurement is an approximated score calculated from 30 disconnected elements (i.e., Sport Australia, 2019). In the United Kingdom and Sweden, physical literacy is measured by a checklist of set capabilities and achievements that every child should achieve (Sport England, 2016), and this is often used to inform assessments in physical education (Lundvall & Tidén, 2013). The measurement methods being used around the world are often reductionist and break physical literacy up into discrete constructs; for a comprehensive investigation into what we mean by reductionist methods and how these are carried out in practice please see in Chapter 13.

An Ecological Dynamics understanding cannot subscribe to reductionist methods of measuring physical literacy as the role of the environment is downplayed in such assessments. One reason for this is that children are asked to complete assessments in environments that are quiet and free from distractions. If we take the concept of motivation, for example, the researcher would sit with the child and complete a questionnaire that is paper-based and ask questions which are broadly related to the child's world but don't attend to their specific context. This is purposefully done in order to tap into a child's thoughts and feelings and the method allows the data to be collected in a manner that enables the research to draw reliable comparisons and conclusions. An Ecological Dynamics conceptualisation of motivation views it as a system property based on the premise of affordances and the environment-child interaction is key. Therefore, if we are to understand and measure motivation in children, we need to observe interactions between the individual and the environment and from this we can build an understanding of aspects of the environment and the tasks that hold value and meaning for an individual child.

8.3 Fundamental Movement Skill as a Measure of Physical Literacy in Children

An enduring focal point for physical literacy measurement has typically been the assessment of fundamental movement skill. It should be noted that fundamental movement skills are not the same as our definition of functional movement skills (see Chapter 2). Fundamental movement skills are defined as observable movement patterns involving the combined use of two or more body parts which include stability (e.g., balancing and twisting), locomotor (e.g., running and jumping) and object-control (e.g., catching and throwing) skills (Logan et al., 2015; Ozmun & Gallahue, 2016;). The term 'fundamental' represents possession of a base of skill competencies that provides the initial building blocks of more advanced, complex movements required to participate (currently and in the future) in various sports, games and physical activities (Seefeldt, Reuschlein & Vogel, 1972; Barnett et al., 2016). Assessment tools to measure movement skills such as the Test of Gross Motor Development are widely used to measure and understand children's movement skills ability. This type of measure provides an insight into a child's basic movement ability and has been reported as both valid and reliable extensively in the literature (Ulrich, 2017).

8.4 The Difference between Fundamental and Functional Movement Skills

The major difference between fundamental and functional definitions of movement is that functional movement skills are predicated on the idea of affordances whilst fundamental movement skills are not. As with the reductionist methods highlighted above for measuring motivation, fundamental movement skill measures give very little consideration to the role of the environment. As was the case with our motivation example, the assessment takes place in closed environments where the assessor asks children to perform a movement skill based on an instruction and a demonstration. The research practice is aligned to the premise that skills are stored in a form of schematic motor programme that a child can recall and execute on demand. From an Ecological Dynamics understanding of movement the lack of affordances regulating behaviour is the key factor that would lead to an impoverished movement skill performance.

8.5 Functional Movement Skill Assessment and Measurement

From an Ecological Dynamics conceptualisation of physical literacy there are a number of important aspects that we must look to incorporate into any measurement of physical literacy. Firstly, it should be affordance based and this requires symmetry between the individual and the environment. This means that the practitioner or assessor should put as much time into their consideration of the environment in which the child is situated as they do into the 'test or task' that they are asking the child to complete. In Chapter 2, we explained that functional movement skills refer to the repertoire of behaviours (cognition, perception and actions) which allow an individual to navigate the environment, interact with others and negotiate tasks to achieve intended goals (Chow et al., 2020). Therefore, if we are to measure functional movement there is a need for the researcher or teacher to have an appreciation of the interactions between living systems, their environments and the reciprocity that has evolved between the two (Kugler & Turvey, 1987). An ecological lens is helpful to comprehend why interactions occur, and more importantly, how these interactions are encouraged (Handford et al., 1997). This is something we will discuss further in Chapter 11 when we outline the Boing project. As practitioners, or researchers, we might begin by observing how children play across a variety of settings, noting down the elements of the environment that they inhabit and engage with. Once we have an understanding of this we can think about how we can nudge the children's explorations to other parts of the environment that will support their development. The analogy that we as human beings would never have realised our ability to swim had the opportunity to interact with water not been forthcoming is an important reflection.

If we are wanting to undertake more formal assessment of a children's functional movement skills, a good place to start is to carefully design an environment that supports exploration and adaptations. After we have created this environment, we need to create conditions where data can be collected reliably and are valid under Ecological Dynamics. This is important, as it is through both authentic and reliable assessment that it will be possible to benchmark and compare across groups of children and to identify children who are most at risk and develop plans to support them. To do this effectively, it is important that children are all given the same opportunities, but that the environment is informationally rich (full of affordances) to invite children to explore (Seifert et al., 2018; Hacques et al., 2020). We also need to consider other important consistent constraints such as children having a set time limit to explore the environment. We may also need to provide prompts to assist with exploration, this may, for example, form open-ended instruction such as asking children: how many different ways can you play with the ball? (Figure 8.1), how many different ways can you travel around the obstacle course? (Figure 8.2) and how many different shapes can you make on, and around, the bench? (Figure 8.3). We should also remember that we want to ensure that the movements are functional. There are two aspects of functionality in this task: the first is to show as many different ways as possible and the second is to respond to constraints set, for example, remember when playing with the ball it must stay inside of the cones (Figure 8.1); when travelling around the obstacle course try not to knock over the equipment (Figure 8.2); when making shapes on the bench don't forget that for each shape, one part of your body should be touching the bench (Figure 8.3).

The next step is to record the children's movement behaviours that you observe. To help practitioners make sense of what they are observing we are required to systematically document the exploration behaviour during movement skill performances. This will

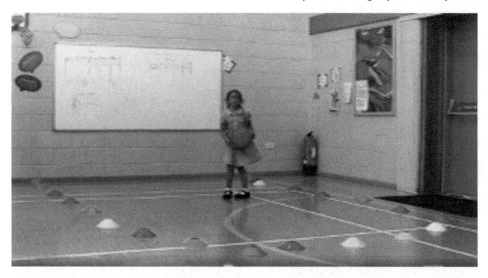

FIGURE 8.1   A child has to find as many different ways to play with the ball as they can but must keep it in the area

allow the practitioner to get an accurate insight into children's functional movement skills and therefore an understanding of their physical literacy. To do this we recommend documenting flexibility and innovation. Flexibility can be recorded by scoring a point each time a new skill is observed in a child's repertoire for the first time during the two minutes. Innovation can be recorded by scoring a point each time a non-original skill is performed innovatively (e.g., in a different direction or using a different body part). Persistence can

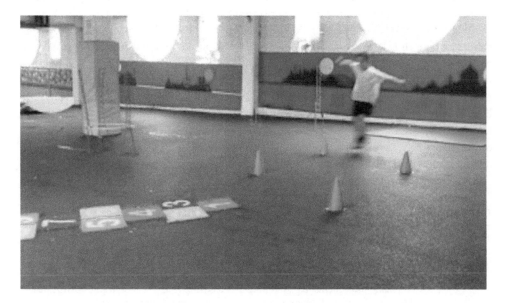

FIGURE 8.2   A child has to find as many different ways to travel around the obstacle course as they can

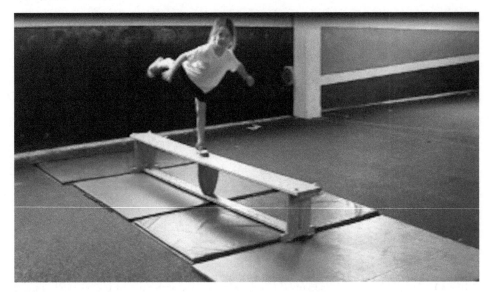

FIGURE 8.3 A child has to find as many different ways to balance on and off the beam as they can

be calculated using the flexibility score divided by the innovation score for each skill. The overall persistence for each child can also be calculated using the total flexibility and total innovative solutions. This gives the practitioner an idea of children's intra-exploration of a movement skill to make it more functional (Table 8.1).

Such an assessment method does not prescribe a technical movement skill template, such as traditional fundamental movement skill measures, but does instead provide an inviting/enriched environment for children to interact with, which enable the practitioner to see children's functional movement skills in all their glory. With a standardised environment and carefully considered task constraints it will be possible to provide reliable and valid data on a child's functional movement skills. It should be noted that, using this form of assessment, a child in a wheelchair can demonstrate a far greater number of functional movement skills based upon their own self-organisation constraints into functional movement solutions than a child who is performing on two feet but has had a poorer physical literacy journey to that point. This is because this assessment is affordance based and therefore individual to the child. It taps into the child's exploration and can be used as a useful measure to progressively understand their physical literacy. To learn more about how to measure functional movement skills and create a rich environment see Chapter 14.

TABLE 8.1 Defining how to measure affordance-based physical literacy assessment

Measurement	*Definition*
Innovation	Total number of different solutions that emerge when performing the same functional movement skill, such as using different body parts to perform similar thematic movements (e.g., jumping 1–2 feet, 2–2 feet, 2–1 foot, using 1 arm, 2 feet)
Flexibility	The total number of different functional movement solutions observed
Persistence	The average number of movement solutions that originate from the same category. Determined by dividing the Flexibility score by the Innovation (also known as Fluency) score

In summary, we have provided an alternative assessment to measure children's movement skills that moves us beyond the current practice of measuring fundamental movement skills that are based on traditional theories of motor learning and do not consider the environment as an important factor in children movement skill performance. We have moved to embrace a functional movement skill assessment that is affordance based and measures through a lens of the child's interaction with the environment. We believe that this type of assessment can provide a better understanding of a child's physical literacy. This assessment can also support researchers in the field of motor development who have been documenting children's low levels of movement skill and its relation to other areas of physical literacy for many years. We believe that functional movement skills assessment is likely to provide more clarity on the quality of movement and other health indicators than the more traditional quantitative measures of physical literacy. We contend that this could provide new insights and improve the strength of relationship between movement variables and other indicators of a child's physical literacy such as moderate to vigorous physical activity.

8.6 Individuality and Intervention

Practitioners such as physical education teachers in schools and coaches at sports clubs are usually given autonomy to design different ways to teach and adapt various pedagogical approaches and practices in order to develop movement competence. However, notwithstanding this, it is the case that assessment and measurement practices shape not only behaviours and how students are assessed but also the way that teachers organise lessons (Chan, Hay & Tinning, 2011; Tolgfors, 2018). It is common in a current youth sport and physical education setting for any form of assessment to have a strong emphasis on ascertaining if learners have acquired a specific movement outcome, with less emphasis on their proficiency at being adaptable in relation to the assessment tasks.

BOX 8.1: RAMIFICATIONS OF FUNDAMENTAL MOVEMENT SKILLS AND FUNCTIONAL MOVEMENT SKILLS ASSESSMENT ON CURRICULUM

Fundamental movement skill assessment

If we are using a static jump as a measure to assess children's fundamental movement skills, then the individual will, more likely than not, focus on practising this, learning to reproduce a jump that will allow them to 'test well'. However, as they are specifying their intention to very specific information, they are unlikely to engage in a meaningful movement experience and instead we are promoting a performative-based curriculum that will not support physical literacy.

Functional movement skills assessment

On the other hand, when adopting a functional movement assessment to assess a child's hopping, the practitioner will need to provide an affordance for hopping. Children can then solve the problems presented in their own unique way (based on effectivities) and it is the way in which the children interact with their environment that will provide the practitioner with insights into their functional movement skills.

Specifically, opportunities to explore individualised movement solutions, which research has shown facilitate the learning of movement competence (Chow, 2013), are downplayed. Whilst there is not a current 'gold' standard for assessing movement competence (Cools et al., 2009; Giblin, Collins & Button, 2014; Ng et al., 2019), assessment rubrics on fundamental movement skills have a tendency to focus on an 'optimal' and 'expected' movement form that limits opportunities for exploration and creativity that could leverage on the individual learner's constraints. A focus on assessing movement competence via the modes of comparison to ideal forms is limiting as it solely focuses on individuals' ability to 'reproduce' movement and neglects the influence of the various constraints (e.g., assessment task) in individuals' movement responses (Seifert et al., 2013; Ng et al., 2019). Crucially, the assessment of a reproduced skill does not provide information about an individual's capacity for adaptability and additionally, may not be functional in relation to the context of the real-world performance-environment (Rudd et al., 2020). We would argue that a Nonlinear- Pedagogy-Based Assessment, such as the functional movement skills assessment discussed in this chapter can help direct teachers to consider designing tasks that encourage exploration and a greater focus on individualised movement solutions. For example, rather than placing an emphasis on an expected movement form that the learners should produce (as an expected learning objective), the outcome could focus on the adaptability and transfer of the movement behaviour to other similar contexts. The emphasis therefore is on the learner's capacity to repeat the outcome though, not necessarily by employing the same pathway to achieve it (i.e., repetition without repetition).

8.7 Summary

At the beginning of this chapter, we set out a conundrum and asked what it means to measure physical literacy. As we have discussed here, there is at present a strong emphasis on non-affordance-based measures of physical literacy across the domains, and particularly in movement competence. We have put forward an alternative proposition that physical literacy measurement across all aspects of physical literacy should be affordance based, and it is our contention that the affordance-based measures of functional movement skill assessment are most valuable in helping us to understand where an individual learner is on their physical literacy journey.

References

Barnett, L. M., Stodden, D., Cohen, K. E., Smith, J. J., Lubans, D. R., Lenoir, M., Iivonen, S., Miller, A. D., Laukkanen, A. & Dudley, D. (2016). Fundamental movement skills: An important focus. *Journal of Teaching in Physical Education*, 35(3), 219–225.

Chan, K., Hay, P. & Tinning, R. (2011). Understanding the pedagogic discourse of assessment in physical education. *Asia-Pacific Journal of Health, Sport and Physical Education*, 2(1), 3–18.

Chow, J. Y. (2013). Nonlinear learning underpinning pedagogy: Evidence, challenges and implications. *Quest*, 65, 469–484. doi:10.1080/00336297.2013.807746.

Chow, J. Y., Davids, K., Shuttleworth, R. & Araújo, D. (2020). Ecological dynamics and transfer from practice to performance in sport. In A. M. Williams & N. Hodges (Eds.), *Skill acquisition in sport: Research, theory and practice*. London: Routledge.

Cools, W., De Martelaer, K., Samaey, C. & Andries, C. (2009). Movement skill assessment of typically developing preschool children: A review of seven movement skill assessment tools. *Journal of Sports Science & Medicine*, 8(2), 154.

Giblin, S., Collins, D. & Button, C. (2014). Physical literacy: Importance, assessment and future directions. *Sports Medicine*, *44*(9), 1177–1184.

Hacques, G., Komar, J., Dicks, M. & Seifert, L. (2020). Exploring to learn and learning to explore. *Psychological Research*. doi:10.1007/s00426-020-01352-x.

Handford, C. H., Davids, K., Bennett, S. & Button, C. (1997). Skill acquisition in sport: Some applications of an evolving practice ecology. *Journal of Sport Science*, *19*(4), 321–349.

Haywood, K. M. & Getchell, N. (2019). *Life Span Motor Development* (7th ed.). Champaign, IL: Human Kinetics.

Kugler, P. N. & Turvey, M. T. (1987). *Information, natural law, and self-assembly of rhythmic movement: theoretical*. Hillside, NJ: Lawrence Erlbaum Associates.

Lingard, R., Thompson, G. & Sellar, S. (2016). National testing from an Australian perspective. In S. Sellar, B. Lingard & G. Thompson (Eds.), National testing in schools: an Australian assessment [Local/Global Issues in Education series] (pp. 1–17). London: Routledge.

Logan, S. W., Webster, E. K., Getchell, N., Pfeiffer, K. A. & Robinson, L. E. (2015). Relationship between fundamental motor skill competence and physical activity during childhood and adolescence: A systematic review. *Kinesiology Review*, *4*(4), 416–426.

Lundvall, S. & Tidén, A. (2013). Assessing embodied knowledge in Swedish PEH: The influence of physical literacy. *ICSSPE Bulletin*, (65). http://urn.kb.se/resolve?urn=urn:nbn:se:gih:diva-3163

Ng, J. L., Button, C., Collins, D., Giblin, S. & Kennedy, G. (2019). Assessing the internal reliability and construct validity of the general movement competence assessment for children. *Journal of Motor Learning and Development*, *1*, 1–20.

Ozmun, J. C. & Gallahue, D. L. (2016). Motor development. *Adapted Physical Education and Sport*, *6*.

Rudd, J. R., Crotti, M., Fitton-Davies, K., O'Callaghan, L., Bardid, F., Utesch, T., Roberts, S., Boddy, L. M., Cronin, C. J. & Knowles, Z. (2020). Skill acquisition methods fostering physical literacy in early-physical education (SAMPLE-PE): Rationale and study protocol for a cluster randomized controlled trial in 5–6-year-old children from deprived areas of North West England. *Frontiers in Psychology*, *11*, 1228.

Seefeldt, V., Reuschlein, S. & Vogel, P. (1972). Sequencing motor skills within the physical education curriculum. *AAPHERD. (EE. UU.). 256p*.

Seifert, L., Strafford, P. B. W., Coughlan, E. K. & Davids, K. (2018). Skill transfer, expertise and talent development: An ecological dynamics perspective. *Movement & Sport Sciences - Science & Motricité*, (102), 39–49.

Seifert, L., Wattebled, L., L'Hermette, M., Bideault, G., Herault, R. & Davids, K. (2013). Skill transfer, affordances and dexterity in different climbing environments. *Human Movement Science*, *32*(6), 1339–1352.

Sport Australia (2019). *The Australian Physical Literacy Framework*. Retrieved from https://www.pescholar.com/wp-content/uploads/2019/08/The-Australian-Physical-Literacy-Framework.pdf

Sport England (2016). *Towards an active nation. Strategy 2016-2021*. Retrieved from https://sportengland-production-files.s3.eu-west-2.amazonaws.com/s3fs-public/sport-england-towards-an-active-nation.pdf

Tolgfors, B. (2018). Different versions of assessment for learning in the subject of physical education. *Physical Education and Sport Pedagogy*, *23*(3), 311–327.

Ulrich, D. A. (2017). Introduction to the special section: Evaluation of the psychometric properties of the TGMD-3. *Journal of Motor Learning and Development*, *5*(1), 1–4.

Way, R., Balyi, I., Trono, C., Harber, V. & Jurbala, P. (2014). *Canadian sport for life-long-term athlete development resource paper 2.0*. Vancouver, Canada: Canadian Sport Institute-Pacific.

9

WHAT WE HAVE LEARNED AND THE WAY FORWARD

James Rudd, Ian Renshaw, Daniel Newcombe,
Geert Savelsbergh, Jia Yi Chow, Will Roberts and Keith Davids

This book has provided an ecological conceptualisation of physical literacy. Re-embracing our ancestry as hunter and gatherers we have started to reveal a way through the sheer scale of socio-cultural constraints that are interacting in the 21st century to challenge the capacity of children in modern societies to live an active lifestyle. As practitioners and educators we have a duty to support children on their physical literacy journey. We now understand that to this aim we must move beyond dualistic and performance-focused pedagogical practices that turn children off from being physically active.

In Section 2 of this book, we introduced contemporary pedagogical approaches such as constraints-led teaching, nonlinear pedagogy, environmental design principles and the athletic skills model which are underpinned by the theoretical framework of Ecological Dynamics. Through careful learning design, these models propose the creation of enriched environments that provide value, meaning and motivation to encourage children to explore and exploit opportunities to interact with the environment. These pedagogical approaches work because they have a fundamental appreciation of how children learn to move. They require practitioners and educators to plan, design and base their judgements and decisions upon children's interactions with the environment and not on a preconceived ideal technique or template movement. An Ecological Dynamics-based pedagogy demands that the educator or practitioner operates at the behavioural scale of analysis with the capacities and dispositions (effectivities) of the child, such as cognitions, preferred ways of moving, emotions and perceptual skills supporting functional movements.

9.1 Physical Literacy Journey

Where the educator or practitioner is able to create an enriched environment which is purposefully designed to provide the feel and freedom experienced with unstructured play, but overlayed with careful learning design, it can provide a powerful platform to support children's physical literacy. Over time, by encouraging children to learn through exploration and allowing them a say in the design of their learning activities, children will develop a deep knowledge of the environment. In these circumstances the educator or practitioner takes on the role of problem setter so that the design is based upon children's functional movement skills and the individual child's capability to detect key and meaningful features of the environment that can be exploited to 'find their way'. It is through these interactions with environment that we will see the emergence of new functional movement skills, that in turn reveal a new knowledge of the environment. This continual process, where value and meaning are associated with affordances in the learning context, leads to an ever-deepening knowledge of the environment. Educators and practitioners adopting nonlinear pedagogical principles and designing environments, such as those outlined in the athletic skills model, will help their students to develop athletic qualities which enable them to quickly reorganise movement systems into relevant coordination patterns that are transferable as they learn which specific behaviours are more functional than others in different play and performance environments. This physical literacy journey is, in essence, wayfinding, an active engagement with the world, seeking, and being constantly responsive to its invitations for re organising actions: whether action is self-navigating from one destination to another, or self-navigating through a movement-related problem during play and physical activity. In all these landscapes, it is the individual's deepening knowledge of the environment that progressively enables them to skillfully interact with the environment. This is how wayfinding can support the ongoing physical literacy journey.

9.2 Physical Literacy in the Community

Over the last three decades, physical literacy has been slowly adopted as a worldwide social movement to support long-term health and well-being of our children and young people. To our knowledge, a growing number of countries are investing in physical literacy and are integrating this into public policy in education and health to help children become more physically active. Whilst this is to be welcomed, it is hoped that countries, and more specifically policymakers, focus less time and energy on creating national top-down prescriptive programmes and shiny new buildings that may not celebrate the cultures of the people residing in the area. Instead, it may be more appropriate to design infrastructure which actively reconnects individuals with the environment such as the Netherlands' widescale application of the athletic skills model across sport and within community spaces.

As we noted in Chapter 3 of this book, physical literacy is rife in the community if we only know where to look. Cage football and street basketball have few associated costs and there is no governing body providing formal rules about who can, and who cannot, participate. Instead, it is an important part of the street culture that supports and teaches young and old and enriches their lives and the lives of others in the community. Too often in developed countries, we believe that the development of new infrastructure and technologies that allow everyone to train and play like the professionals they see on TV will make sports participation more attractive and generate a more physically active population. However, as we have learned, new facilities which are disconnected from the community, and technologies that attempt to shortcut the learning journey, are unlikely to have an impact. Rather, investing in policies that promote wayfinding will support a deeper knowledge of the environment leading to a deeper understanding of the performer/performance environment.

9.3 Opportunities in Physical Literacy Measurement

In a growing number of countries, where physical literacy has been integrated into policy, we are seeing an increasing interest in how it can be measured. Whilst measurement is undoubtedly an important pedagogical tool, if this is intended to inform practice, we need to be mindful about how we can best use measurement and assessment to capture a child's physical literacy. Current practice focuses on reductionist approaches where children perform isolated assessment tasks, with each measure being a different construct of physical literacy. As we highlighted in Chapter 8, none of the measurements tools currently being used are affordance-based, that is, they are asymmetrical in that they focus on the individual but pay little attention to the environment in which the learner is situated. We discussed in Chapter 14, some of the exciting new Ecological Dynamics-based assessments that are being designed around the premise of affordances whilst still providing rich data about children's functional movement skills in the forms of movement creativity. We do, however, have to be careful both at a national level and at a school and class level, that we do not slip back into a performance-based pedagogy, or curriculum, where the sole focus is on developing a prescribed motor technique at the expense of supporting children to develop wayfinding skills within their local environment.

9.4 Here We Offer Some Ideas and Recommendations for How We can Prioritise Play in the 21st Century to Support Children's Physical Literacy

9.4.1 Recommendation 1: After-School Care Should be Re-Defined as 'After-School Play'

The growing trend for parents to work and children to attend after-school care programmes is unlikely to change. However, rather than reducing the levels of physical activity, this can present an opportunity as the provision of after-school care is a fertile place for children to be given the freedom and space to have fun, express themselves and explore their own movement capabilities. Too often commercially-driven (that is, adult-led) programmes do not have the knowledge or skills to move beyond a babysitting service or a 'throw the ball out' approach. As recommended by the AAP report (Yogman et al., 2018) see Chapter 1, there is a need for children to have more opportunities to engage in self-regulated activities which provide a variety of purposeful experiences leading to spontaneous activities which harness the imagination, which can be *invited* by play settings such as school playgrounds. Here, we propose that such environments could play an important role in the enrichment of an individual's physical literacy. Chapters 1–3 provided an ecological rationale suggesting that enrichment activities are those which support participants to interact with challenging environments which have just enough uncertainty and variability to engage in playful activities requiring the pick-up of information to solve problems and make decisions expressed in actions. However, to achieve these goals administrators responsible for appointing after-school club operators need a more nuanced understanding of physical literacy and the ways in which commercial operators can offer schools and children an environment that supports inquiry, exploration and learning.

9.4.2 Recommendations 2: Promote Play in Local Parks

Perhaps, a silver lining of the COVID-19 crisis in 2020 was the significant increase in spontaneous inter-generational play activities that emerged when schools were closed. Children have an inherent desire to get out of the home, exercise, play and have fun. Perhaps, local councils can embrace this opportunity by investing in more local, attractive non-symmetrical parks and play facilities that invite families to explore and interact with them. The design of playscapes could provide various opportunities for social, emotional, perceptual, cognitive and physical enrichment. Additionally, programmes that encourage and provide facilities to support safe community backyard games in the locality of children's homes could be developed. Indeed, this 'hands-off supervision' may encourage parents to allow their children to 'come home' to play.

9.4.3 Recommendations 3: Play into Coaching and Teaching

As revealed in Chapter 3, competitive, backyard games promote the conditions to facilitate the development of holistic physical literacy skills and we, therefore, propose that they should become a key feature of talent development programmes. At time, facilities should be made available to allow young children to just play (Orlick & Botterill, 1975) and perhaps one session per week can be put aside to enable children to play without being constantly corrected and 'coached'. In support of this, we suggest that the session should be treated as an 'event' that is emotionally engaging and memorable. These events should be organised and run by the children themselves (Cooper, 2010), but a framework should also be offered. For example, the time length of games should be kept short to allow maximal participation for all, they should be encouraged to manipulate rules to cater for all participants of different abilities and no game should ever be allowed to become one-sided. In order to maximise engagement and promote as many learning opportunities as possible, we recommend keeping team numbers small, so play lots of small-sided games rather than one big one. Playing areas and equipment should be designed based on the concept of affordances and be carefully body-scaled and matched to the action capabilities of children. Flair, cheekiness, innovation and creativity should be encouraged, celebrated and rewarded. However, this does not have to be via formal rewards but could simply be a general chorus of 'olé' (for example), if a footballer managed to beat a defender with a unique solution, or a basketballer added a twist to a lay-up or shot.

Competition is important in providing the catalyst for learning and should be carefully designed into events; however, we strongly support inclusion, but also that fairness means provided opportunities for individuals to display their talents and not be humiliated. Rules should, therefore, be flexible and sensitive to this requirement. The use of 'ladders' instead of round-robin leagues is one way of ensuring that individuals or teams play against opponents of similar abilities. Handicapping is also a recommended way of providing challenges for 'better' players whilst at the same time allowing young or weaker players the opportunity to test themselves. At times we suggest that children should be presented with problems that are difficult to solve. Such tasks will help the practitioner to get a feel for how an individual reacts when it 'gets hard' and can help promote the ubiquitous quality of 'grit' (although we would prefer to talk about perseverance and focus more on how to support the development of problem-solving skills)! Finally, we would encourage practitioners to remember that becoming good takes a long time and to help children achieve excellence requires engaging in the activity for a significant sustained period of time. Consequently, the overall goal should be to create environments which *invite* children to 'fall in love' with the sport (see the impact of street basketball – Chapter 3) which will also potentially lead to promoting a lifelong engagement with their chosen games.

References

Cooper, R. J. (2000). The impact of child abuse on children's play: A conceptual model. *Occupational Therapy, 7,* 25–276. doi:10.1002/oti.127

Orlick, T. & Botterill, C. (1975). *Every kid can win.* Chicago, IL: Nelson Hall.

Yogman, M., Garner, A., Hutchinson, J., Hirsh-Pasek, K., Golinkoff, R. M. & Committee on Psychosocial Aspects of Child and Family Health, & Council on Communications and Media. (2018). The power of play: A pediatric role in enhancing development in young children. *Pediatrics, 142*(3), 1–17.

SECTION IV

Exploring New Avenues of Research to Understand Physical Literacy

Section 4: Introduction

The adoption of the theory of Ecological Dynamics as a means of developing a comprehensive roadmap to conceptualise and operationalise physical literacy is in its infancy and consequently, there are limited examples of researchers or practitioners adopting the ideas in their work. However, a few pioneers have embraced the challenge and are starting to grapple with the real-world demands we encounter when applying great theoretical ideas in messy 'real-world' environments for the first time. As we have highlighted in this book we believe that currently the focus of research is too heavily skewed towards the measurement whilst too little attention is paid to the actual implementation, including exploring the thoughts of school staff, practitioners and children. We would also argue that there needs to be a clear focus by researchers on understanding the fidelity of pedagogical delivery.

In that context, in Section 4, the final section of this book, we present a series of Case Studies that will spotlight the work of researchers and practitioners who have 'put themselves out there'. These case studies explore innovative methods for measuring, develop new pedagogical approaches and seek to understand the impact of these on the wider community. Each case study provides exemplars as to how the ideas of nonlinear pedagogy (NLP) and Environmental Design Principles are being used in practice to enhance the physical literacy of populations as diverse as primary and secondary physical education in schools, dance education (see Chapters 10 and 11), implementation of NLP and Constraints-Led Approaches in high-performance sport (Chapter 12). A particularly challenging task is how to assess physical literacy when the working definition of what physical literacy is in an Ecological Dynamics approach is so different to the traditionally held views and reductionist measurement methods currently in vogue (Chapters 13 and 14). We would argue that the value in assessing physical literacy from an Ecological Dynamics approach is in the practitioner taking the time to observe and understand where each individual learner is on their physical literacy journey and to consider how this might be enhanced through active design. We recognise that this practice is in its infancy and is not perfect, but this is not a reason not to do it. All of these case studies attempt to articulate and demonstrate how research across the globe is reconnecting with the original intentions of physical literacy with contemporary pedagogical under an Ecological Dynamics rationale.

10

PHYSICAL EDUCATION

Combining Movement Education and Nonlinear Pedagogy to Provide Meaningful Physical Education Experiences

James Rudd, Katie Fitton Davies, Laura O'Callaghan, Matteo Crotti, Rachael Grace and Lawrence Foweather

10.1 Introduction

Across the world, physical education (PE) aims to enhance functional movement skills during early childhood (United Nations Educational, Scientific, and Culture Organisation, 2013). For the last ten years in Liverpool, England, we have been monitoring children's movement skills and wider physical activity levels and have found that children who attend pre-school in areas of high deprivation score very low on children's movement skill assessments and, as they get older, this leads to a diminished physical literacy journey which is associated with lower health outcomes later in childhood (Foulkes et al., 2015; McWhannell et al., 2018). In view of this, we decided to try to support these children and help them catch up during their first year of primary school and Dr James Rudd and Dr Lawrence Foweather devised a research programme called The *Skill Acquisition Methods fostering Physical Literacy in Early-Physical Education (SAMPLE-PE)*.

The aim of the SAMPLE-PE project was to consider the efficacy of reintroducing movement education curriculums to enhance children's functional movement skills. These curriculums advocate that children should experience a broad curriculum of dance, gymnastics and team games taught in a way that promote versatile exploration throughout the PE lesson with the teacher promoting inquiry-led and discovery-based learning methods. These curriculums went out of fashion in the 1970s because it was thought that they were too complex as there was no clear delivery method and teachers, therefore, had to use their own experiential knowledge to make decisions regarding implementation and delivery. For many teachers, particularly those at primary school level, who had more limited training in delivering PE than their secondary-based PE colleagues, these challenges seemed simply beyond them. Subsequently, movement education was replaced by health-related fitness and skill-based performance sport pedagogical approaches. In this chapter we provide a case study which presents dance and gymnastics lessons for young children. These lessons incorporate elements of a nonlinear pedagogy and movement education and are compared with more traditional linear PE lessons in gymnastics and dance. We conclude the chapter by explaining the approach of the SAMPLE-PE project.

10.2 Example 1: Dance for Young Children

10.2.1 Linear Dance

Dance is a popular element of the curriculum, particularly in primary schools where poor facilities often limit PE activities. Dance requires little more than an empty 'school hall' with minimal levels of equipment. In primary school dance lessons, we typically see the teacher leading from the front of the class modelling the movements of a pre-planned choreographed dance whilst the children copy the teacher's movements in time with the music. As the children begin to memorise the dance, the focus of the teacher is on correcting movement errors when the reproduction of the movements strays away from the 'correct' movement model. The requirement that all children 'dance' in the same way can lead to slow, repetitive progress as often children struggle to remember the connected sequences or produce the movements as required. An important consequence of this approach is often low levels of motivation with children having minimal levels of autonomy, perceptions of their own competence and relatedness to each other and the teacher (Chow et al., 2015).

10.2.2 Nonlinear Pedagogy to Support Movement Education Dance Curriculum in Young Children

In contrast, movement education offers a creative dance curriculum, where the sessions' goals are not based on children reproducing specific dance movements, but rather, to provide opportunities for personal expression through dance. Nonlinear pedagogy includes a number of principles: representativeness, manipulation of constraints, attentional focus, functional variability and the maintenance of pertinent information-movement couplings through task simplification, and these, with thoughtful integration, can provide a framework and guide for movement education lessons and support children in acquiring a broad range of functional movement skills through dance. The practitioner is able to introduce previous meaningful experiences from the classroom that all children have knowledge of, this could, for example, be a storybook they have read together, or it could be a topic they have covered in class. Thanks to this shared previous experience the dance practitioner can help the children to create enriched environments within the lesson through the use of their imaginations. There are many benefits of this approach that align to physical literacy; for example, there is a natural goodness of fit because by using their imaginations children create a world that they can inhabit and explore whilst the practitioner gently guides and exploits the emergence of new functional movement solutions. An example of using experiences from a classroom activity that invite creative dance movement might be when children have been learning about garden bugs, a typical activity in primary schools. The dance teacher may set up the lesson space as an imaginary garden and use animals found there, such as the caterpillar and the butterfly to stimulate children's thinking about the contrasting ways these animals move. They can then bring these movements to life in their own way with the teacher supporting exploration. In this example, children's imaginations are being employed in a similar way to the way that we saw Native Americans unlock the effectivities (Gibson, 1979: skills, predispositions, capacities) of the animals they embodied and therefore were able to perceive things that they could not perceive in their human form. The teacher can further exploit this imaginative imagery through the manipulation of constraints such as the tempo, beat or volume of the music to afford new learning opportunities. Additionally, task constraints that can be used to increase the task complexity include introducing equipment such as ribbons or balls or changing the environmental constraints by moving the lesson from indoors to outdoors. By manipulating the learning landscape and limiting verbal instructions, the teacher is able to move from being the focal point driving the lesson, as was the case in our linear example, to becoming a facilitator, allowing the children to guide the emergence of their own learning. The net effect of these principles is to provide the children with greater autonomy, increased perceptions of competence and improved relatedness, as this approach encourages them to regulate their own behaviours and to experiment to find solutions that best answer their own individual needs within the given context. In summary, this pedagogy promotes a strong sense of self-regulation and creative movement behaviours commensurate with each child's current action capabilities.

10.3 Example – Gymnastics for Young Children

10.3.1 Linear Gymnastics

In traditional primary school gymnastics lessons, the teacher will typically structure sessions to follow the format of a warm-up and then move on to learning basic foundation movements such as forward and backward rolls, handstands, headstands and cartwheels before moving on to combining sequences. Similar to a traditional games lesson, most of these 'basics' are taught using 'decomposed' tasks with high levels of prescriptive instruction. For example, when teaching a forward roll to stand, children are taught using prescriptive instructions such as '*start in a squat on the balls of your feet with knees together. Place your hands flat on the floor with spread hands. Whilst maintaining pressure on your hands, tuck your head and place the back of your head between your hands whilst pushing with your legs to roll over forward. Maintain a rounded back by contracting your abs, and keep looking at your knees. As you roll forward, try to maintain momentum to roll up onto your feet and stand up without pushing off the floor with your hands. Your arms should just reach forward at the end of the roll.*' If the children master this, the teacher will deem it safe to introduce equipment; for example, getting the children to perform a forward roll on a bench, and the final part of the lesson will involve each child performing what they have learned to the rest of the class. This linear approach to gymnastics assumes that children all have the same capacities/effectivities and that breaking the skill into components and then mastering each of these in isolation will equip all the children to perform the skill, in this case the forward roll, safely.

10.3.2 Movement Education and Nonlinear Pedagogy Gymnastics

The nonlinear pedagogy gymnastics lesson adopts a similar approach to that used in the dance lesson and is built on the teacher encouraging the children to use their imaginations to create movements that demonstrate a goodness of fit between their current action capabilities and the task demands. This approach supports the exploration of an individualised enriched environment that is unique to each child. Again, similar to the approach used in dance, storytelling is a favoured stimulus. In England, typically, in the first year of schooling, children read the storybook, *The Gruffalo* (Donaldson, 1999), which tells the story of a mouse's walk through the woods and to protect himself from being eaten by a number of large and dangerous animals who inhabit the woods, he invents a fictional monster called the Gruffalo. This book is much loved by children and it is therefore easy for teachers to incorporate the world of the Gruffalo into PE lessons thus building on the children's experience of the story and unleashing their imaginations. Recreating a learning environment that simulates that found in the woods enables the teacher to create an abundance of affordances (e.g., flora and fauna) that the teacher can exploit to support the emergence of new functional movement skills. For example, children are encouraged to adopt the movements of the characters in the book. The character of the snake is used to support rolling, and through embodying the effectivities of a snake, the children move their bodies close to the floor, slithering and sliding as they traverse under, over and around equipment. Other characters from the book allow contrasting opportunities for movement. For example, the owl is used as metaphor to help children explore being on top of the equipment and movements such as leaping and jumping emerge naturally without direction from the teacher. Through careful questioning, the teacher can further encourage functional movement solutions to emerge by proposing new analogies such as 'can you roll like a mouse down a hill?' or 'can you roll like the Gruffalo playing in the stream?' These manipulations are made at the teacher's discretion, however, it is important that the teacher understands that in this type of lesson, in contrast to the linear lesson, it is acceptable, even highly desirable, for children to display different movement solutions to the same task and that regression in skill is inevitable when altering constraints (such as equipment). As long as the skill demonstrated is functional and it achieves the outcome then it is acceptable.

10.4 An Exemplar of Movement Education Lesson with the Integration of Nonlinear Pedagogical Principles

In each gymnastics lesson within the nonlinear pedagogy curriculum, all equipment is set out prior to the lesson and remains out throughout the duration of each lesson and, importantly, the teacher does not prescribe the type of skill to be learned – such as forward roll. Instead, the teacher uses equipment that will invite behaviours such as rolling, for example, designing lots of slopes in the environment by placing wedges and other equipment at angles which encourages children to explore different ways to roll based upon their own effectivities. By designing this specific environment, the teacher provides the children with novel experiences that create invitations to use gravity to learn to roll. To develop functional and adaptive movements, the teacher creates mini-games within the lessons, and employs teaching methods such as analogies and questions. For example, within the gymnastics rolling lesson, children play a game where they become the snake in the book who has to move treasure (beanbags) from one side of the water (the mat/floor) to the other. The treasure cannot get wet (so they need to keep the beanbag off the mat/floor), and each piece of treasure must be rolled across the water in a different way, otherwise the Gruffalo might spot them. These types of activities create an external attention of focus, and at the heart of the activity is problem-solving that requires functional movements solutions. The teacher is able to make decisions on what task constraints to manipulate, based upon their observations of the children's, for example, where a child demonstrates a stable and functional motor skill, the teacher will act to destabilise the skill by altering task constraints or changing the task goal. In the example of the snake in the gymnastics rolling lesson, the teacher creates instability in movement by giving the children different types of equipment (treasure) to transport (i.e., different size, shape, weight) across the mat. This could involve changing the treasure from a beanbag to a football that will lead to self-organisation and the emergence of a new functional movement solution. Another option could be for the teacher to ask the child to play the game on a new area of the play space, such as on one of the slopes, as this will again require self-organisation and result in the emergence of new functional movement solutions. Changing these task constraints will result in new affordances. In contrast to a linear approach, the teacher must also keep in mind that as long as the skill is functional and achieves the outcome of the lesson then it is to be accepted.

10.5 The SAMPLE-PE Research Project

Designing movement education curriculums to explore how PE lessons can best support physical literacy in young children was an integral aspect of the SAMPLE-PE project. Our approach was to create and compare linear and nonlinear lessons and then to evaluate the impact of these pedagogies on children's development. This project also moved the area of fundamental movement skill research forward in a number of ways. First, a protocol paper was published setting out what we were aiming to do and how we would go about it (Rudd et al, 2020 [https://www.frontiersin.org/articles/10.3389/fpsyg.2020.01228/full]). As can be seen in the protocol we included novel assessments to understand children's functional movement skills (not just fundamental movement skills). The project also had a comprehensive process evaluation where we listened to the voices of the stakeholders (teachers, headteachers, teacher and children), and additionally, we examined the fidelity of the pedagogical delivery. Whilst such an approach was hugely time consuming it did allow us to learn objectively what had worked, what we needed to rethink and how best to move forward.

References

Chow, J. Y., Davids, K., Button, C. & Renshaw, I. (2015). Nonlinear pedagogy in skill acquisition: An introduction. New York, NY: Routledge.

Donaldson, J. (1999). *The gruffalo*. Oxford: MacMillan Children's Books. (ISBN 0-333-71093-2).

Foulkes, J. D., Knowles, Z. R., Fairclough, S. J., Stratton, G., O'dwyer, M., Ridgers, N. D. & Foweather, L. (2015). Fundamental movement skills of preschool children in Northwest England. *Perceptual Motor Skills*, *121* (1), 260–283. ISSN 0031-5125.

Gibson, J. J. (1979). The ecological approach to visual perception. Boston, MA, US: Houghton, Mifflin and Company.

McWhannell, N., Foweather, L., Graves, L. E. F., Henaghan, J. L., Ridgers, N. D. & Stratton, G. (2018). From surveillance to intervention: Overview and baseline findings for the active City of Liverpool active schools and SportsLinx (a-CLASS) project. *International Journal of Environmental Research and Public Health*. Mar 23; *15*(4), 582. doi: 10.3390/ijerph15040582. PMID: 30720781; PMCID: PMC5923624.

Rudd JR, Crotti M, Fitton-Davies K, O'Callaghan L, Bardid F, Utesch T, Roberts S, Boddy LM, Cronin CJ, Knowles Z, Foulkes J, Watson PM, Pesce C, Button C, Lubans DR, Buszard T, Walsh B and Foweather L (2020) Skill Acquisition Methods Fostering Physical Literacy in Early-Physical Education (SAMPLE-PE): Rationale and Study Protocol for a Cluster Randomized Controlled Trial in 5 -6-Year-Old Children From Deprived Areas of North West England. Front. Psychol. 11:1228. doi: 10.3389/fpsyg.2020.01228

11

BOING AND PHYSICAL LITERACY

A Play-Based Movement Programme for Community, School and Sport

Will Roberts, Danny Newcombe, Sean Longhurst, Kit Cutter and Ben Franks

11.1 Introduction

This case study offers an overview of a research project currently being undertaken at the University of Gloucestershire and Oxford Brookes University (United Kingdom). Our aim is to support practitioners to create playful, active and inclusive practice that promotes the development of physical literacy in community, school and sport settings. In order to design purposeful, playful and rich environments, there is a need for practitioners to appreciate the reciprocity between a learner and their environment (Kugler & Turvey, 1987). This *individual-environment fit*, as we introduced in Chapter 2, allows us to consider how engagement with the environment will invite or *afford* movement solutions. This fundamental premise has allowed us as a team to consider the purposeful design of playful environments that act as a vehicle to support the journey of a child's physical literacy development. The use of the term journey is one that we are cautious about, as far from suggesting an end point or destination to be reached, we are merely suggesting that young people's learning experience is akin to the wayfinding experiences previously discussed in this book. We wanted to encourage problem-solving through various inclusive, engaging and motivating activities; therefore, as a team of academics, we developed what we called the Playtank (an online resource of playful environments and delivery materials called playgames) based on foundational principles. Our founding idea was that if our students (at the time based at Oxford Brookes University) could focus on the pedagogy of supporting their learners, rather than spending all their time planning lessons, then we could truly accelerate their practice in-situ. We developed a realisation that utilising a nonlinear pedagogical approach, underpinned by an Ecological Dynamics framework, would allow us to design a rich landscape of affordances, inviting individuals to engage with an array of movement possibilities to support their physical literacy journey. It has allowed us to create learning environments that are poised on the edge of chaos but that can be tweaked by practitioners before and during sessions to manage the instability (i.e., chaos) to promote learning. The rules of a game, the size of the area, the number of children on each team and the amount and size of equipment available were all manipulated to create environments that offer the opportunities aligned to the chosen developmental focus of the practitioner and/or children. As we have progressed, the Boing project has matured into one where we are engaging in the practitioner landscape by designing workshops for practitioner educational purposes as well as supporting the development of *playgames* to support practitioners as they engage young people

11.1.1 Boing: A Play-Based Curriculum to Nurture Physical Literacy Through Active Play

As we have suggested earlier in the book, physical literacy can be embedded (i.e., via direct perception and self-organisation) and embodied (i.e., information specified by our perceptual systems and capabilities). This interaction with the environment is key to finding movement solutions to problems posed in sport, physical activity or physical education settings. Bernstein (1967, p. 228) defined the ability to solve emerging motor problems (such as a new game, movement or a complex problem in our case) as *dexterity* and suggested that a need for flexibility is key in skill development to encourage learners to seek solutions to the same or similar motor problems. With this in mind, we have been focused on developing playful games for primary aged children through a Sport England funded project called *Boing* (more information can be found at www.boingkids.co.uk). As part of this project, we have advocated that practitioners design variability into their activities and set appropriate problems for learners. In this project, we designed a series of 130 playgames (our name for the games we have designed), utilising an Ecological Dynamics framework to promote the endowment of physical literacy (Roberts, Newcombe & Davids, 2019). In our design, we suggested that when designing practice tasks, practitioners should utilise 6 key principles to engage their learners through play, namely:

1. Practitioners as environment designers
2. Affordance driven practice design
3. Manipulation of constraints
4. Co-adaption and collaboration
5. Managed chaos
6. Dexterity and degeneracy

The integration of these principles in designing practice tasks provides a framework to support the embedding of theoretical tenets of Ecological Dynamics into practice. In essence, we have attempted to operationalise theory in practice for coaches and teachers in their context. It is important to note that no one principle is viewed by us as having more importance than any of the others. Furthermore, it is essential that these principles are employed as a guide and not a prescriptive set of rules, provided with the purpose of supporting practitioners with the tools to be the architects of their learning environments.

11.1.1.1 Principle 1: Practitioners as Environment Designers

In this section, we outline the importance of carefully designed environments. Whilst we have developed a number of environments as part of the Boing project, a key evolution to these playgames is that of encouraging practitioners to manipulate the game to meet the needs of the individuals in their context (see Figure 11.1). We have been careful to attend to the development of a learner's physical literacy in our design of playgames by providing carefully designed environments which offer an array of affordances for each specific group with which we worked. We have been able to work with over 700 coaches and teachers and a range of partners to support the development of the project and we are committed to the idea that the learning environment facilitates problem-solving which in turn shapes the movement solutions of the learners (see Figure 11.2). Observing the

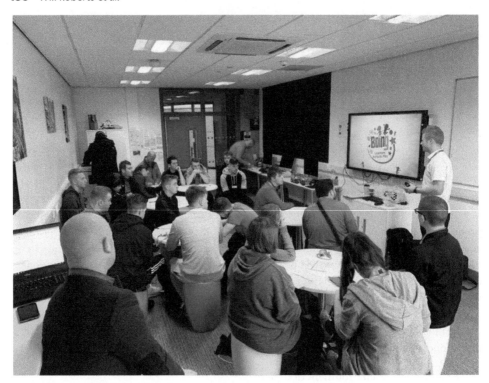

FIGURE 11.1 Boing workshop supporting the development of Boing principles

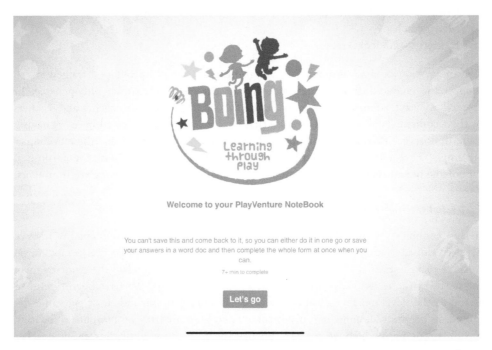

FIGURE 11.2 The online playventure: an interactive approach to supporting practitioner development

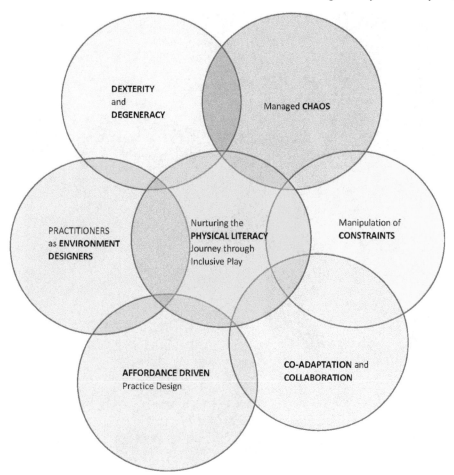

FIGURE 11.3 Principles for practice design to nurture the physical literacy journey for practitioners (Adapted from Roberts et al., 2019)

children engaged in decision-making is a positive sign, as we believe they are more likely to be exploring their own development across many different domains (e.g., their physical, emotional or social development) when immersed in solution finding (see earlier discussions on wayfinding). If we are to attend to the holistic development of children, it is important to embrace the embodied nature of physical literacy (see Figure 11.3). Thus, it is important to ensure that the decisions of *when, why* and *how* to act are invited through the interactions with the environment and not directly by the teacher or coach. If we are supporting children to, for example, develop and realise their ability to hop and balance using a single leg landing then we need to provide an environment that facilitates the development of this understanding. For instance, in the *Bears in the Woods* playgame (visit www.boingplaytank.co.uk/playgame-bearsinthewoods; see Figures 11.4 and 11.5), the task constraints are manipulated to encourage stepping, jumping or hopping from one disc to another carefully placing the discs so that we can challenge an understanding of which distances invite hopping and which do not as a function of the variable distances

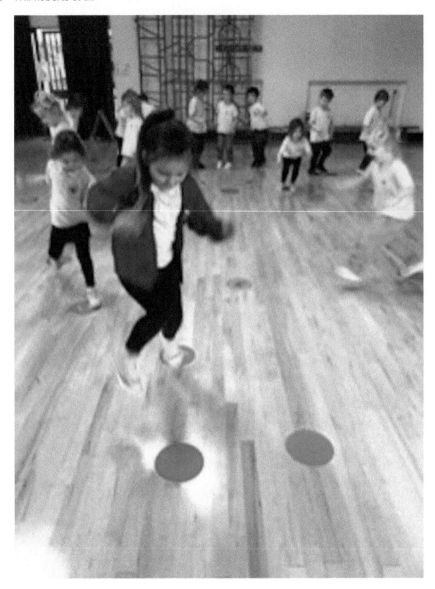

FIGURE 11.4 Some primary aged children playing *Bears in the Woods*

between spots. Further, the encouragement to move from spot to spot in time with the beat of a drum is an example of inviting functional movement through task constraint manipulation. Success within the environment is characterised by increased self-realisation which is evident in more efficient and strategic routes being planned and executed by the children. Practitioners must therefore carefully consider the ways in which learning environments are designed. In doing so, practitioners can ensure learners find themselves immersed in appropriately challenging, yet achievable activities that promote high levels of perceived competence.

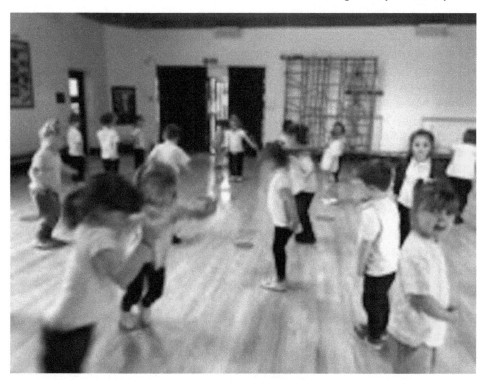

FIGURE 11.5 Children will plot their route through *Bears in the Woods* and find their own way to jump and land depending on their capabilities

11.1.1.2 Principle 2: Affordance Driven Practice Design

When designing-in affordances into the playgames, the essential question practitioners must ask is '*does the environment offer, invite and/or encourage learners to explore the opportunities for action related to the current development focus?*' For example, it might be that we want to develop weight transfer, or balance, or deceleration. Designing learning tasks through the manipulation of constraints to provide affordances for action requires practitioners to be 'problem setters' who are able to implicitly invite desired perception-action couplings. The *Affordance Driven* principle proposes that the actions are shaped through the learner exploring the relevant landscape of affordances in the environment. So, if we want to develop deceleration (as an example of a physical development focus), then we would need to design a landscape that requires speed to be high with some demand for acceleration (small end zones, or challenging obstacles at high speed where change of direction is needed). The ability to act upon an appropriate affordance at any one moment is a key part of learning to play and solve problems with effective movement solutions. It is vital to consider that recognising when to act (*perception*) is as important as the movement itself (*action*) and the two must remain coupled to the learning environment. Just because an affordance is available does not mean an individual should use it and knowing when a learner 'ought' to use an available affordance is perhaps just as important as knowing how to use it (Heft, 2003). We might, for example, set an obstacle course or set of challenges which are not 'standardised' and ask learners to move around in the quickest way, but not in a pre-ordained or predictive order. Encouraging a learner in this example to try and search for the best solution, trialling different routes and exploring movement, acceleration and deceleration that is based as much on decision making as it is movement capability. A playgame we have developed that encourages this type of practice is Tik Tok (www.boingplaytank.co.uk/playgame-ticktock), which has a course, and a series of 'taggers' to encourage variability and changes in speed, movement direction. In our playgame, the learner negotiates the traffic of other children as well as set structures. In simple terms, well-structured environment design must offer learners the opportunity to move beyond 'what' they must do, and towards an understanding that allows them to construct for themselves the 'how, why, where and when' of movement. In essence, we need to ask if the answer that the problem elicits regarding the decisions and movements of an individual is the intention of that specific environment.

11.1.1.3 Principle 3: Manipulation of Constraints

If we understand which affordances within the landscape are most inviting for a group of children, we will be able to manipulate key constraints in a learning environment to support learners in searching for and discovering, effective solutions to a movement problem. Practitioners can manipulate constraints to shift the learner's intentions, to support the development of new bodily attributes (e.g., increased muscle strength, flexibility, postural stability), to improve motor skills or through promoting on-going perceptual learning to increase differentiation. The ability to learn to act upon the most appropriate affordance at any one moment is a key part of learning to play games; however, in their desire to focus practice there is often a temptation by coaches and teachers to over-constrain practice by introducing rules or restrictions to explicitly *force* 'desired' actions (see Renshaw et al., 2019 for a discussion on avoiding the over constraining trap). It is therefore imperative that practitioners do not just consider which constraints are manipulated, but also how and why they are embedded in the learning environment. Examples of poor practice include practices such as the 'you must make 5 passes before scoring' rule often seen in invasion games. This type of constraint over-emphasises the mere reproduction of an action and misses the key point in invasion games: that learners need to understand the function of a pass to a teammate and perhaps what other opportunities to act there are in an environment. The simple manipulation of task constraints allowed us to encourage multiple editions of the same problem to occur within the one environment. For example, in the *Dragon Catching* environment, a game based on 'capture the flag,' we can increase the width of the access point by ensuring there are multiple *dragons* to defend and capture. An interesting observation of this in practice is that the learners will migrate to the iteration of the game they feel most comfortable engaging with, which evidences self-realisation in action.

11.1.1.4 Principle 4: Co-adaptation and Collaboration

Principle number four is based on the notion of collaboration. We have seen in our playgames that children working together is important when nurturing and promoting physical literacy beyond physical competence and towards a more holistic understanding of the concept as espoused in this book. On the Boing project, it has been important for us to support learners in developing an understanding of how their interaction with others within the environment can impact on both their own development, and upon others. These important pro-social and psychological aspects of development have been integral to the project given the range of contexts we have been working in. To do this, we have developed a number of our playgames that move the emphasis from individual competition onto collaboration. The presence of affordances that promote collaboration can be an important aspect of exploration for young people. For example, in our playgame Chain Tag (see www.boingplaytank.co.uk/playgame-chaintag) we have observed that children are beginning to take note of others learners capabilities (whether they are quicker, slower, stronger, taller, better or worse decision makers) because success is predicated on being able to move and problem solve together. We have observed in Boing sessions that a learner's interactions with others within an environment can have a significant impact on exploring inherent self-organisation tendencies. This continuous process has been characterised as co-adaptation. With each learner's behaviours constrained by the information from the actions of the other learners in the environment (Passos, Araujo & Davids, 2016) there are opportunities to shape behaviour with carefully designed practices focused on collaboration and co-adaptation. Practitioners should avoid setting problems for learners to solve in environments devoid of other learners. Task constraints must be manipulated to provide learners with the opportunity to collaborate and co-adapt. For example, the environment created by the *Chain Tag* playgame is an example of how a game based on the rules of the traditional *tag* game can be adapted and manipulated to focus on collaboration. In this game, players are expected to join together in order to form a chain and cannot separate the chain in order to tag others. This can be adapted in many of the games where joining learners up as pairs in any of the games provides an increased emphasis on collaboration as well as being a useful method for differentiation as seen in Figure 11.6.

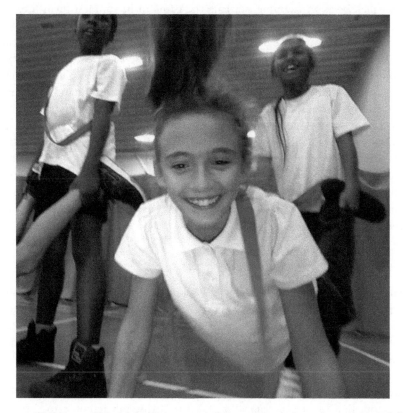

FIGURE 11.6 Children collaborating in a game of *Space Rangers* in order to successfully solve the game

11.1.1.5 Principle 5: Managed Chaos

Bowes and Jones (2006) discussed the notion that complex systems are open to fluctuations and consist of complex chaotic behaviours. Put simply, the learners in the practice environment will endeavour to make sense of the chaos they are presented with by interacting with the task constraints by intentional and goal-directed means. This leads us to the deliberate manipulation of control parameters (via task constraints) to move individuals into less stable areas and create these phase transitions (Handford et al., 1997). It is proposed that if a system is poised at the edge of chaos (at a point where there are many solutions available) it has the ability to create emergent problem-resolving behaviours (Langton, 1990). This tipping point on the edge of chaos is a location of instability for learners, which is useful in facilitating exploration of different movement solutions. If a system is located in a region which is too stable, then the resultant behaviours may be accordingly static, with little demand made on the inherent pattern forming system tendencies. In contrast, any system that is located in a region which is always too unstable will become inherently chaotic and unmanageable (Davids et al., 2003). If the designed practice task is not capable of providing opportunities for learners to resolve consistent questions, then the system may be too chaotic. Furthermore, if a novice learner is placed into an environment with a large number of other learners who are also searching for their own performance outcomes, the information at a localised level could become too difficult to perceive and act upon. If we take *Escape the Zoo* as an example, starting the game in its simplest form (i.e., starting the game with all learners being zoo animals to collect food from the wild) will help manage the information flows perceived by these learners. The practitioner can then add task constraints (i.e., adding a zookeeper) to increase the level of instability in the game. To help find the balance between stability and instability, we need the children engaged in constant and active play. In order to facilitate constant and active play, we aimed to design environments that are more continuous and self-generating in nature, where the teacher is not needed to initiate the start and the finish of the active period. This has been achieved through the manipulation of task constraints to create environments that regenerate on an infinite, continuous loop. The design of environments where the instability in the system is constantly shifting is based on the notion that complex systems exhibit tendencies towards stability and instability, supporting learners in continuously (re)organising in response to a constellation of available constraints (Renshaw et al., 2010).

11.1.1.6 Principle 6: Dexterity and Degeneracy

Bernstein (1967, p. 228) defined dexterity as the ability to find a motor solution to solve any emerging motor problem functionally, quickly, rationally and resourcefully. He identified the need for flexibility in skill development to encourage learners to seek different solutions to the same or similar problems, thus advocating the need for practice task design to incorporate variability into learning contexts. In neurobiology, this is known as exploring system *degeneracy* (Edelman & Gally, 2001). In movement behaviour, degeneracy supports the greater flexibility, adaptability and robustness needed for a learner's functionality during task completion. *Repetition without repetition* is Bernstein's response to the perceived oversimplification within the traditional model for skill acquisition and the inclusion of

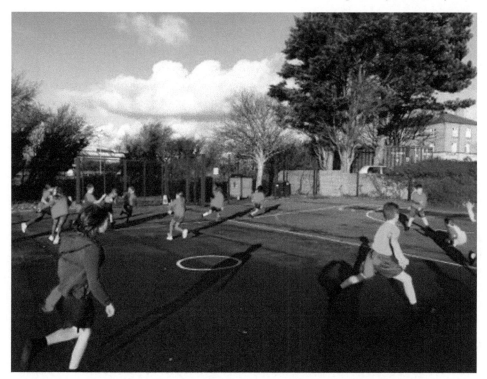

FIGURE 11.7   A game of *Escape the Zoo* that is poised on the edge of chaos, offering an abundance of movement possibilities

variability. Providing environments which allow lots of problem-solving opportunities is essential in allowing learners to repeatedly search and explore effective adaptable movement solutions. The presence of functional variability is a hallmark of more skilled performers (Davids, Bennett & Newell, 2006) and the generation of functionally variable movement patterns is an important characteristic of skilled learners operating within a dynamic environment. As a result, manipulation of task constraints in practice environments must offer both repetition and variation to facilitate this process (Travassos et al., 2012). Practitioners can purposely manipulate task constraints to increase the variability. Taking *Tidy my Room* as an example, this is achieved by increasing the number of rooms, the number of people in each room or the size, weight, surface, colour – of equipment. In summary, learners need to be provided with task constraints that allow them to explore dexterity in their interactions with the performance environment. Another example can be seen in Figure 11.7.

11.2 Summary

In summary, we have attempted to address some specific challenges that our undergraduate students were facing in their pedagogy of coaching the individual. Taking away some of the time to plan and organise sessions allowed us to focus on their development as practitioners in being able to teach or coach young people using an Ecological Dynamics framework whilst adopting a nonlinear pedagogy to nurture physical literacy. Importantly, this afforded us the opportunity to understand some of the challenges in developing truly nonlinear approaches to developing physical literacy as it forced us to face the realities of developing the whole person and not just focusing on skill acquisition. By approaching the development of physical literacy through the design of purposeful environments, developed on the six principles of Boing, we have seen an emergent understanding of movement activity of which has given us some of the evidential and empirical basis to confidently support practitioner education through our funded Sport England project. Adopting an ecological lens is helpful to comprehend why interactions occur and more importantly how these are encouraged (Handford et al., 1997). Most pertinent to these is the recognition of the importance of affordances, which are defined by Gibson (1967) as opportunities for action provided by the environment or ecology, we exist in. Understanding that affordances are environmental properties (Gibson quoted in Weiss & Haber, 1999, p. 129) available as resources for the individual that can be utilised to regulate behaviour (Silva et al., 2014) has been central to the design of Boing's *playgames*. We would urge researchers and practitioners to utilise the free website to access the Boing playgames and begin to critically engage in thinking about how we might nurture the physical literacy journey.

References

Bernstein, N.A. (1967). *The control and regulation of movements*. London: Pergamon Press.

Bowes, I. & Jones, R. L. (2006). Working at the edge of chaos: Understanding coaching as a complex, interpersonal system. *The Sport Psychologist, 20*(2), 235–245.

Davids, K., Bennett, S. & Newell, K. (2006). *Movement system variability*. Champaign, IL: Human Kinetics.

Davids, K., Glazier, P., Araujo, D. & Bartlett, R. (2003). Movement systems as dynamical systems. *Sports Medicine, 33*(4), 245–260.

Edelman, G. M. & Gally, J. A. (2001). Degeneracy and complexity in biological systems *Biological Sciences – Evolution, 98*(24), 13763–13768.

Gibson, J. J. (1967). In E. G. Boring & G. Lindzey (Eds.), *History of psychology in autobiography* (127–143). New York, NY: Appleton-Century-Crofts.

Handford, C. H., Davids, K., Bennett, S. & Button, C. (1997). Skill acquisition in sport: Some applications of an evolving practice ecology. *Journal of Sport Science, 19*(4), 321–349.

Heft, H. (2003). Affordances, dynamic experience, and the challenge of reification. *Ecological Psychology, 15*(2), 149–180.

Kugler, P. N. & Turvey, M. T. (1987). *Information, natural law, and self-assembly of rhythmic movement: Theoretical*. Hillsdale, NJ: Lawrence Erlbaum Associates.

Langton, C. R. (1990). Computation at the edge of chaos: Phase transitions and emergent computation. *Physica D, 42*, 12–37.

Partington, M. & Cushion, C. (2013). An investigation of the practice activities and coaching behaviors of professional top-level youth soccer coaches. *Medicine and Science in Sports, 23*(3), 374–382.

Passos, P., Araujo, D. & Davids, K. (2016). *Competitiveness and the process of co-adaptation in team sport performance*. Frontiers in Psychology, 10(7), 1562. 1–5.

Renshaw, I., Chow, J. Y., Davids, K. & Hammond, J. (2010). A constraints-led perspective to understanding skill acquisition and game play: A basis for integration of motor learning theory and physical education praxis? *Physical Education and Sport Pedagogy, 15*(2), 117–137.

Renshaw, I., Davids, K., Newcombe, D. & Roberts, W. (2019). *The constraints led approach: Principles for sports coaching and practice design*. London: Routledge.

Roberts, W. M., Newcombe, D. J. & Davids, K. (2019). Application of a constraints-led approach to pedagogy in schools: Embarking on a journey to nurture physical literacy in primary physical education. *Physical Education and Sport Pedagogy*, *24*(2), 162–175.

Silva, P., Travassos, B., Vilar, L., Aguiar, P., Davids, K., Araújo, D. & Garganta, J. (2014). Numerical relations and skill level constrain co-adaptive behaviors of agents in sports teams. *PloS One*, *9*(9), 107–112.

Travassos, B., Duarte, R., Vilar, L., Davids, K. & Araújo., D. (2012). Practice task design in team sports: Representativeness enhanced by increasing opportunities for action. *Journal of Sports Sciences*, *30*(13), 1447–1454.

Weiss, G. & Haber, H. F. (1999). *Perspectives on embodiment: The intersections of nature and culture*. London: Routledge.

12

HIGH PERFORMERS

Physical Literacy Is Still an
Important Consideration

Ian Renshaw, Danny Newcombe and Will Roberts

12.1 Backyard Cricket: The Nursery of Australian Cricket

12.1.1 Introduction

For over 150 years, informal games of cricket have been a staple pastime for Australian youth and families and have acted as a task vehicle for the holistic physical literacy for which Australians are renowned. As identified in Chapter 1, play is considered essential for optimal child development and many young Australians choose the task vehicle of cricket as their preferred form of play and by default the development of their physical literacy. The love and cultural importance of cricket in the lives of Australians has resulted in numerous hours of play (i.e., 'practice'). Playing fields were easily accessible in the accommodating climate encouraging effortlessly amassed hours of participation and subsequent skill development. Cricket mattered, and this was reflected in huge numbers of children participating in the sport, often trying to emulate the signature moves of their heroes. When not playing, every chance was taken to watch local 'grade' cricket as state and Australian players regularly turned out in these games. Heroes are important, and impromptu games would often spontaneously emerge on the boundary edge or on the outfield during breaks in play (see Chapter 1) and just like the young basketballers of New York City, local heroes were accessible and observable. The knock-on effect on motivation for these youngsters cannot be under-estimated as they knew that being from 'round here' could result in you playing for your state or country. Indeed, the 'talent pathways' were quite simple to understand and until more recent times, the idea that a player, playing first-grade cricket was only ever two good innings away from playing for Australia was still taken for a truism. When they couldn't get to games, youngsters followed games through listening on the 'wireless' and eventually watching on television.

For a cricket-loving nation, every spare moment was viewed as an opportunity to indulge in their passion. For example, family gatherings or days at the beach often involved setting up cross-generational games that could last all day and night with adults joining and leaving games as other duties (chatting to grandma, making dinner or fetching more beer) were fulfilled. Whilst collectively known as backyard games, all Game rules and local environmental constraints shaped the emergent effectivities of youngsters. Just like pick-up basketball in New York (see Chapter 3), backyard cricket has many forms and can be played alone or by two or more players. Games are not limited to the backyard though, and can be played on streets, playgrounds, in gaps between buildings, beaches, waste ground, driveways or even in corridors inside buildings. Below we discuss how the unique interaction of individual, task and environmental constraints provided opportunities for holistic physical literacy to be acquired subconsciously through daily play activities (see Chapter 1).

12.2 The Games

The unique affordances of each game venue were highly significant in underpinning the intentions, emotional regulation and skill sets of young players and had a strong influence on the way they played the game later in their careers. For example, famously, the world's greatest ever batsman, Don Bradman, who was brought up in country New South Wales, spent hours hitting a golf ball against a water tank with a stump, with these constraints shaping his unique grip, stance and backlift. The example of Bradman is typical of many Australian greats as described in Steve Cannane's (2009) excellent book, *First Tests: Great Australian Cricketers and the Backyards That Made Them*. Local rules were always unique to the individuals playing the games but are also shaped by the constraints of the physical environment in which they are played. For example, a 'six and out' rule was often enforced to discourage players from hitting the ball into a neighbour's garden or onto a dangerous road. Sometimes, the ball had to be hit along the ground to avoid breaking windows or hit in specific directions as walls or other features limited hitting in those areas. Often the surfaces games were played on had a major impact on the emergence of strengths and weaknesses as well as other aspects of physical literacy such as balance or learning to deal with sub-optimal conditions. For example, Neil Harvey, a great left-handed batter for Australia in the 1960s, played much of his backyard cricket on the cobblestoned streets around his home in the backstreets of Sydney. Consequently, as the ball would deviate significantly once it bounced, he used his feet and tried to hit the ball before it hit the ground. Harvey credits this environmental constraint as being the key reason why he was never stumped in test cricket when playing for Australia (Cannane, 2009). On a psychological level, learning to play in non-symmetrical or more variable environments created adaptable players who were not phased when conditions were unfavourable later in their careers (Renshaw & Chappell, 2010). For bowlers, run-ups had to be fitted in around features such as greenhouses (e.g., former England swing bowler Matthew Hoggard; Hoggard, 2010), whilst batters used trees and fences to invite shots in particular directions (e.g., Matthew Hayden – see https://www.youtube.com/watch?v=Pcxgr1CYu2Q). A more recent non-Australian player whose unique bowling style was shaped by his environment was Makhaya Ntini of South Africa, who learned to bowl on artificial pitches laid on concrete. The key challenge for Ntini was that he had been given a set of bowling boots with spikes (sprigs in Australian language) and this meant he could not stand up on the concrete. He, therefore, bowled wide of the stumps and this became his signature method years later when playing for South Africa. His unique angle of attack gave him a significant point of difference to other more orthodox bowlers and made him very difficult to bat against as batters were not attuned to the unique ball flights. When children played backyard games, bats were often improvised and made from simple pieces of wood; old bats cut down in length or width or even miniature, autograph bats were utilised. Balls could be tennis or table tennis balls or even scrunched up balls of paper if a hard cricket ball was not affordable or appropriate to the play environment. Wickets could be made from dustbins or chalked onto walls of garages or sheds. When played by children, before or after school or in holidays, teams would be matched to be equal as there were no age categories. To cater for size and skill differences, rules were adapted, so younger children had a decent chance and older more skilled players were not allowed to dominate games.

12.3 Backyard Games as the Nursery for Greatness

Whilst backyard games were played for fun, they have also been described as the true academy of Australian cricket as they allow players to devote hours of holistic practice where they developed unique skills, mental skills and the physical conditioning that underpinned their later expertise (Cannane, 2009: Renshaw & Chappell, 2010). Backyard games also promoted holistic physical literacy as 'unstructured' children's play-based activities (Roberts, Newcombe & Davids, 2019; Button et al., 2020) enriched relevant behaviours including perceiving information, coordinating actions, making decisions, cooperating with others in groups and teams, working to achieve intended actions, solving problems and emotionally regulating behaviours under different conditions in life (Renshaw & Chappell, 2010).

Perhaps the key characteristic of backyard cricket is that it provided experiences that cultivated a 'romance' with cricket and a lifelong love of the game (Bloom & Sosniak, 1985). Motivation is a key construct in Whitehead's (2013) conception of physical literacy (see Chapter 2), and here we argue that backyard games resulted in high levels of self-determined or intrinsic motivation necessary to sustain individuals through the ups and downs associated with the journey to high-level performance. Longevity in playing cricket is more likely to occur if these early experiences take place in fun-based activities without pressure from over-bearing adults; sadly, a feature of many formal play environments experienced by youngsters who are playing organised cricket games at earlier and earlier ages. The key goal of backyard cricket in-line with all play was and (and is) having fun and this aligns neatly with the views of expert players and coaches who believe that the primary focus for young cricketers should be on fun and enjoyment and general skill development through simply taking part (Phillips et al., 2014). Those who showed a true passion for the game were suggested to be most likely to continue into the investment phase.

As highlighted above, backyard cricket has been viewed as a significant socio-cultural constraint in the emergence of many of the great Australian players from Victor Trumper to Mike Hussey (Cannane, 2009) and often, the unique environments of individual's early experiences underpin the emergence of playing styles that are often the later signatures of experts (see Cannane, 2009). As former Australian great Matthew Hayden says 'I firmly believe that every backyard shapes someone's destiny'. A keen advocate of the natural ways of learning via backyard games is former Australian Cricket Centre of Excellence Head Coach Greg Chappell who strongly believes that these early experiences in backyard sports are a significant factor in providing a foundation upon which expertise can develop (Renshaw & Chappell, 2010, p. 156):

> I mean those early years of where we played our make believe test matches in the back yard or whether we were an older brother or younger brother or whether it was just me throwing the ball against the wall, the imagination was a really important part of it as well and I think many years later I used that experience in visualization sessions and so on.

Just like Hayden, Chappell is a firm believer that these early experiences are a significant factor in providing a foundation upon which expertise can develop. As Chappell notes, after playing backyard cricket against his older brother (Ian, a future Australian captain), the mental demands of test cricket were 'a breeze' (Cannane, 2009)!

12.4 Empirical Evidence

12.4.1 Batting

Research has provided support for the role of unstructured cricket games in the journeys of future elite cricketers. For example, Weissensteiner et al. (2008) looked at the developmental histories of skilled and unskilled batsmen and found that by U-15, skilled batters who had played for their states had taken part in three times the amount of unstructured practice as their non-skilled counterparts (see Figure 12.1).

12.4.2 Fast Bowling

In terms of fast bowling, identifying the conditions that underpin the emergence of fast bowling is of significant importance for those responsible for designing talent pathways as possessing outstanding fast bowlers is crucial to team success in international cricket. The role of the fast bowler is to be the spearhead of a team's attempt to bowl out the opposition and is the most physically and mentally demanding task in cricket as well as demanding a high level of skill. Traditionally, Australia has produced many great fast bowlers, and the harsh climate that produces hard and fast pitches that rewards fast bowling has been thought to be a significant factor. However, to get a more detailed picture of the key factors

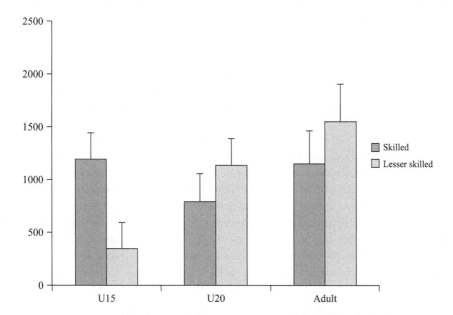

FIGURE 12.1 The total number of hours accumulated in unorganised cricket activity was also greater for the highly skilled players in the U-15 age group (adapted from Weissensteiner et al., 2008)

underpinning the development of expert fast bowlers, Phillips et al. (2014) interviewed 11 past or present Australian international elite fast bowlers who had taken more than 2,400 international test wickets in over 630 international test matches. This group were truly elite with all of them having taken at least 75 international test wickets and appearing in at least 20 international test matches. In terms of the early experiences, unstructured practice activities were found to be important, with 73% of experts saying that they did not specialise in fast bowling until the late teens. Several experts were not even involved in structured cricket until late in their teens. This factor highlights the danger of early specialisation and highlights that a particular advantage of late specialisation for future fast bowlers was that it limits their exposure to injury associated with high bowling workloads during maturation. In Australia (and the United Kingdom), representative and school pro-grammes result in heavy workloads around the key ages of 14–16 and many young bowlers are at risk of back injuries. All experts mentioned the importance of 'backyard' cricket in their development which was often undertaken with siblings and friends in unstructured environments allowing skill development in all aspects of the game, and with a strong focus on enjoyment, participation and competition.

12.5 What Can We Learn from Backyard Cricket for Contemporary Coaching?

Given that the evidence provides strong support for backyard games as being extremely influential in the development of expert cricketers, why are we seeing fewer and fewer youngsters playing them? A key challenge is that the majority of early cricket experiences are provided in formal programmes in clubs and schools. Quite simply, there is insuf-ficient time for young players to play informally. The lack of explorative, spontaneous, meaningful, imaginative and purposeful play experiences is being noticed by coaches who are concerned that young players lack 'game sense' as well as wider physical literacy skills as highlighted by Whitehead (2013), as highlighted in Chapter 2. Backyard games give youngsters the opportunity to undertake enough 'practice' to capitalise on one's movement potential; learn to adapt to asymmetric environments moving with poise, economy and confidence; being perceptive in reading all aspects of the environment and responding to the possibilities of movement; having an established sense of oneself as an embodied being and finally having an understanding of the qualities of one's own movement performance.

The 'limitations' of the contemporary cricket learning environments has resulted in coaches searching for new ways to 'coach' up and coming young players. One new method-ology currently being adopted across many development and high-performance programmes is the constraint-led approach (CLA) (Renshaw, Davids & Savelsbergh, 2010) which has been shown to be more effective in developing the batting skills of emerging cricketers than a more traditional drill-based approach (Connor et al., 2018). A key tool in using CLA in cricket coaching was the development of the Battle Zone. We introduce the Battle Zone next and describe how the AIS/Cricket Australia Academy developed and embraced this new approach to cricket coaching and put it front and central in their programme.

12.6 Bringing the Backyard Game into the 21st Century: The Battle Zone

A key goal of Greg Chappell when he became Head Coach at the AIS/Cricket Australia Academy in 2009 was to find ways of creating better learning than that found in nets and

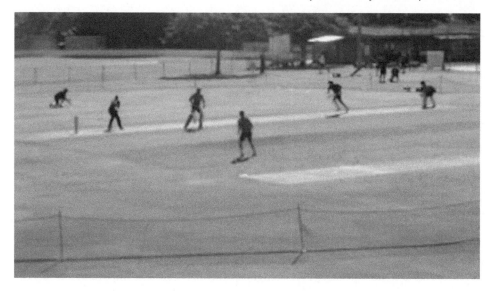

FIGURE 12.2 The Battle Zone. A net is placed around the one-day fielding circle and once stepping into the playing arena, the player is in a 'battle'

in emotionless centre wicket practice. At the time I (Renshaw) was working with the coaches and we came up with the idea of recreating match intensity by putting a low 'net' on the 30-m circle. Our key goal was that when playing a 'practice' game, the players needed to be constantly challenged and engaged emotionally, mentally and physically in the practice tasks. We, therefore, christened the practice area the 'Battle Zone'. The layout of the Battle Zone can be seen in Figure 12.2. It should be clear that the Battle Zone is as much a concept as it is a physical space. It is based on adopting all the principles of the CLA and in particular with creating affective learning design to recreate the intentions, emotions and information-movement coupling commensurate with real games of cricket (Renshaw et al., 2010; Headrick et al., 2015).

The Battle Zone puts the player at the centre of the learning process and requires each player to take responsibility for his or her own learning. It provides practice that enables transfer of skills to the real game and can help players to learn to solve problems on the run. Typical Battle Zone sessions are co-created by the coach and player(s) based on current rate limiters which can include technical, tactical mental or physical factors. Games are designed by manipulating constraints to facilitate the opportunity for the player to explore new ways of overcoming the weaknesses. For example, if a spin bowler needs to improve his ability to bowl on turning pitches, coaches can 'doctor' the playing surface to create turn and bounce. If the player is a poor decision maker when fatigued conditions can be created that require the player to perform in this state (see Renshaw & Chappell, 2010 for an example how we have achieved this in a practice session).

In summary, the Battle Zone shifts the control back to the players, allowing them autonomy and enhances their feelings of competence as it enables them to gain vital experiences that are representative of real match conditions. It allows coaches to target specific rate limiters of individual players by matching game design to their needs. Importantly, the Battle Zone concept is built on playing 'real' games and captures cricketer's love of competition. Players reported that practicing in a Battle Zone game was much more valuable than simply having a net or a centre wicket practice. The approach is very much like backyard games and is much more fun for both players and coaches. Similarly, we believe it is just as effective and can be described as the 21st-century backyard game.

12.7 International Field Hockey

12.7.1 Daniel Newcombe and Will Roberts

This case study is centred around the international field hockey context that one of the authors (Daniel Newcombe, DN) is situated within. The aim of this case study is to build on Chapter 6 where we explored the idea that practitioners are architects of their environment to provide a rich example of how the coaching team employ and understanding of nonlinear pedagogy (NLP) and how we also ensure that the physical literacy of the international athletes is attended to within the programme design. More specifically, the case study will provide an exemplar of how we facilitate the players' ability to develop an embedded and embodied relationship with the performance environment. We will explore how the coaches use performance analysis data to identify targeted areas for improvement and subsequently reverse engineer the emergence of important affordances in the landscape to enhance the players' ability to wayfind in the performance environment through emergent functional movement skills. The team DN coaches is currently ranked in the top 20 international teams in the world (18th in the current Federation International Hockey world rankings) and takes part in regular international tournaments on a European, Commonwealth and World level. The squad is made up of approximately 30 players, all aged between 17 and 30 years. The majority of the players operate as part-time or semi-professional hockey players, requiring them to balance work, domestic and international hockey commitments. On average, the group has between 50 and 60 contact days per year. The training contact time is mostly 'camp' based, comprising 4 × 2-hour training sessions across two-day periods. Additionally, the team is brought together approximately four to six days prior to each major tournament. The group is working hard to build on its recent, significant, improvement with the goal of continuing to narrow the gap between the current level of performance and that of the leading teams in the world. When designing a curriculum, we consider multiple facets of each athlete and treat them as a person first. Their mental well-being and health, their knowledge of and about their own performance and supporting their emotional development are equally as important as developing their performance. The curriculum we design and practices we employ are a crucial part of this bridging process. To simplify this section, where appropriate, it will be written from the first-person perspective of DN and the coaching team.

> **Coach Reflection** – *Within our international hockey context, we have previously fallen into the trap of providing generic environments that lack specific purpose and any form of targeted development. We have found that investing time at the start of the design process, establishing the key intentions within our curriculum provides us with the guiding light we need to design an effective curriculum.*

In line with every other top team in the world, the team has access to a performance analyst who records and collects data on each game. In the following section, we explore

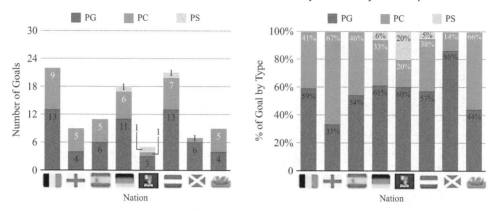

FIGURE 12.3 Depicts the number of goals scored by each team and the method by which they were scored (Meyers & Rowe, 2020)

how the Welsh coaching team utilises data in the curriculum design process. The following statistics and infographics provide an excellent overview and analysis of the performance data from all the fixtures at a recent high-ranking tournament (Myers & Rowe, 2020). The analysis provides a complete set of performance outcomes achieved by all teams throughout the tournament. The data promote a comparison between the side DN coaches and the other teams in the competition. As can be observed in the data, there are significant points of difference between the Welsh team and the higher-ranked teams, highlighting the key phases of the game we need to focus on and align specific intentions to being more successful within them. From this analysis we can reverse engineer the relevant available affordances and ensure they are designed-in to the curriculum. This will often include affective development as well as physical. For example, we might apply pressure (scoreboard, crowd, purposefully poor refereeing decisions) to the players to support their intentional interaction with emotional affordances. Significant credit needs to go to Sam Rowe (Hockey Wales, Analyst) and Laura Myers (Sports Consultant) for their work in providing the analysis to inform this process.

In Figure 12.3, we can see the number of goals scored by each team and the method by which they scored them. You will not be surprised to find that the teams finishing in the top half of the tournament scored significantly more goals than those finishing in the lower half. That insight we probably did not need the data for. However, understanding how these teams generate the opportunities to score more goals may provide us with useful insight and direction for our curriculum.

Interestingly we can see that it took an average of 11 circle entries, seven circle possessions and four outcomes to score a goal (Figure 12.4). A circle entry is recorded every time the ball enters the attacking circle situated around the goal. The laws of the game dictate that a goal can only be scored if a member of the attacking team contacts ball in the attacking circle. This magnifies the significance of earning circle possessions, which are recorded when an attacker touches the ball in the circle. An outcome is recorded if the attacking team manages to manufacture a shooting opportunity, penalty corner or penalty stroke from the circle possession. A more physical literate team will become more attuned and develop the ability to effectively interact with, the affordances present in the performance environment (Araújo & Davids, 2011). Put simply, we are interested in how often we can facilitate

11.1 Entries per Goal Scored				**6.9** Possessions per Goal Scored				**4.3** Outcomes per Goal Scored		
	AJT	DEF			AJT	DEF			AJT	DEF
	8.7	47.5			5.7	30.0			3.2	21.0
	15.8	14.1			11.3	7.4			6.7	3.7
	11.3	9.8			6.1	5.7			4.1	3.7
	9.8	11.5			6.7	6.0			5.0	4.6
	25.6	7.7			14.0	5.2			7.6	3.4
	9.3	17.7			5.7	10.0			4.0	6.4
	11.4	9.3			6.0	6.9			3.1	4.0
	10.0	9.8			5.8	6.0			3.4	3.6

FIGURE 12.4 Provides an overview of the team's circle efficiency throughout the tournament. The data include the number of goals scored per circle entry, circle possession and outcome

possession of the ball into the attacking circle and manufacture an outcome. If we compare the data from the Welsh team to that of the leading teams in the tournament, we can see that circle efficiency compares favourably and we can reason that once the ball enters the attacking circle and the team is in possession, they generate a similar ratio of the goals of that of the top teams. We can also deduce that the team produces a good number of goals per outcome. These data made us feel confident about the players' ability to convert circle possessions into goals and thus we predict that by increasing the supply (more circle possession) we would in turn score more goals. This insight is further supported by looking at the circle possession data, we earnt well below half (52) the amount of circle possessions the leading teams generated, all of which manufactured over 120 circle possessions across the tournament.

The information provided so far does not equip us with anything specific enough to help us design our curriculum, however, it does provide us with useful context and a starting point for further exploration. We decided to dig into the data further as we attempt to locate the critical phases and the associated affordances we would need to design-in to the practice environments. Some useful insight can be gleaned from Figure 12.5, it is interesting that the majority of goals scored at the tournament (72%) were a product of the defending team regaining possession high up the pitch (Zone 3 or Zone 4). Furthermore, exploring the data we found a clear correlation between how many times a team won the ball back in Zones 3 & 4 and the number of circle possessions generated. This understanding led us to overarching intention for our next training block – winning the ball back higher up the pitch (Zone 3 & 4).

Interestingly, the method of gaining possession in the build-up to a goal can be seen in the detail provided in the graph below (Figure 12.6). Somewhat surprisingly to the coaching team, we can see that possession earnt from either a Free Hit, Interception or Tackle led to 75% of goals scored in the tournament. All of these methods of possession regain can be classed as live turnovers, more specifically turnovers that happen in live play and allow the team who have gained possession to attack against a disorganised defensive system, with a reduced number of defenders between themselves and the goal. This provides us with some really useful insight and informs some of the constraint manipulation outlined

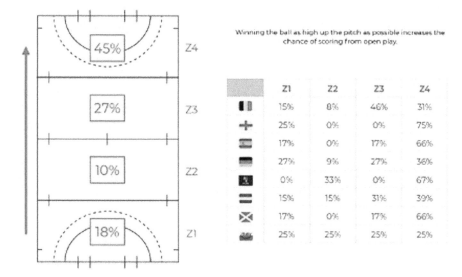

FIGURE 12.5 Provides the location where possession of the ball was gained by the attacking team in the build-up to a goal

in the curriculum design section. As a coaching team, it is important for us to consider the holistic conceptualisation of physical literacy. This encourages us to explore the interacting elements and the impact these will have on the players engagement with the affordances. For example, we have often overlooked the motivation and confidence elements on the players interaction with the environment.

It is through this analysis that we arrive at our intention for our next training block, 'to increase the number of live turnovers in Zones 3 & 4'. A task easier said than done within the context of international field hockey. In order to win the ball back higher up the pitch

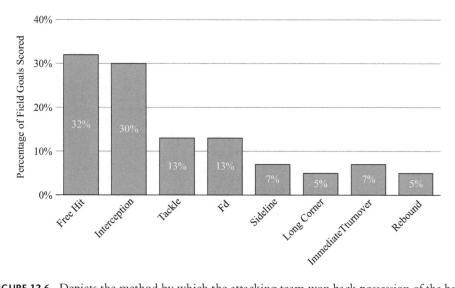

FIGURE 12.6 Depicts the method by which the attacking team won back possession of the ball in the build-up to a goal

the defensive team must aggressively commit a large number of players to Zones 3 & 4. It is therefore essential that the playing group develop a clear understanding of the risk-reward associated with this challenge. Whilst the rewards of winning the ball back higher up the pitch are high, the risk of conceding a goal also in turn dramatically increased. Such aggressive pressing has the potential to leave our defensive system stretched and as a result venerable to penetration, a product of pressing aggressively requires us to defend a significantly bigger playing area. Hence, developing a collective understanding of how, when and most importantly when not to apply this tactic will be crucial to our success. Furthermore, the importance of developing the players individual actions that will allow us to contain the ball in the desired area of the pitch and generate the live turnover should not be underestimated. In the following section we will explore how the Constrain to Afford principle is applied to design the curriculum to meet the training block intention. As identified in Chapter 6, this principle promotes a subtler, somewhat indirect and more patient approach. The desired actions are certainly encouraged and, indeed, solicited by the practice design to develop a more embedded and embodied relationship with the environment.

12.8 The Training Block

The training block outlined below consists of three separate training camps designed in preparation for upcoming international fixtures. All three camps are two days in length, and each is comprised of 4×2-hour training sessions. Designing effective training environments is achieved by the coach manipulating the appropriate task constraints, a practice, which on the face of it appears to be a relatively simple undertaking. However, as we have presented in Chapter 6, the rationale for decisions made within the curriculum are often complex and nuanced. The following section provides an outline of the key task constraint manipulations we plan to employ across the three training camps. We will explore the impact these manipulations will have on the affordance landscape and the players anticipated interaction with them. We find it useful to use a constraints builder as a guide for this process (Renshaw et al., 2019), it prompts us to consider which constraints to manipulate where, when and most importantly why (Figure 12.7).

TASK

Boundaries, Size and
Shape of Pitch
Scoring – Size, Shape and
Orientation of Goals
Players – Number and
Team Allocation
Player Start Position
Ball Feed Position
Point Scoring System
Time Limit
Additional Rules and
Regulations
Equipment Modifications

FIGURE 12.7 Shows the task constraint elements from the environment builder we consider when designing our environments (adapted from Renshaw et al., 2019)

The initial phase of *task* constraint manipulation is what we have termed 'organising our furniture', we feel it is essential to ensure we have the base of our practice designed prior to considering further manipulations. In this phase we carefully consider the *boundaries* (size and shape of pitch) of our training environments and the position of our *goals* (type, number and orientation) within them. In the first training camp, we made the decision to provide smaller scaled environments (relative to the number of players). We anticipated that the smaller scaled environments will in essence ensure the players are in closer proximity and subsequently reduce the risks associated with pressing aggressively. These smaller scaled environments will therefore *offer* the players an increased number of opportunities to press aggressively in attempting to generate *live* turnovers higher up the pitch. It is hoped that the increased number of opportunities to press (the designed-in affordance) will increase the number of opportunities for individual players to engage in individual tackle situations and interceptions and thus meet the intention of the first training camp. There is an attempt by the coaching team to design-in affordances that facilitate the holistic development of the athletes' physical literacy. A crucial element that will need to develop is the physicality required to press aggressively, this requires us to delicately position the size of the playing area to overload these demands. In the second training camp, we will increase the relative size of the training environments. The subsequent increase in playing area will require the players to be more selective about when, and when not to press aggressively and thus reduce the number of opportunities to press aggressively. However, it is important to consider the *trade-off* associated with this decision. Whilst there is the potential for less opportunities to press, the adjusted affordances landscape will create the need for the pressing team to work collectively in order to keep the ball in the designated area of the pitch. Any errors in collective positioning, individual body positions or tackling technique will result in the attacking team being able to *play-out* of this area and attack against an unstructured, underloaded defensive system. Whilst we may get less opportunities to press, it is likely to promote more effective solutions when these instances do occur. In the third and final training camp, we will really exaggerate the size of the playing area(s). This increase in space will require the defending team to employ appropriate systems of play and strategies to engineer an opportunity to press aggressively. The adjusted affordance landscape will facilitate the need for players to *execute* the more tactical elements we wish to develop within the third training camp. We made the decision to maintain a traditional goal position (*scoring*) throughout the three training camps. We debated adjusting the goal positions for a significant period; however, we felt that the positive impact on the affordances in relation to the intention would be negligible and as a result the loss of representation (RLD) associated with adjusting them wasn't worth the trade-off.

Coach Reflection – *Within our performance curriculum we aim to spend the significant amount of time at or just over thus tipping point, with such limited contact time we need to maximise any opportunities for learning and development. It has taken a whilst for us as coaches (and even longer for the playing group) to feel comfortable with experiencing errors within our practice environment and reframing them if not as a positive sign, or at the very least an opportunity to learn.*

The next *task* constraint we consider is the *players (number and team allocation)*. In the first training camp, we chose to keep the player numbers on each team relatively small (4v4–5v5). By keeping the player numbers small we predict an increase in the number of interactions in and around the ball for each individual. The smaller *player* numbers combined with tighter pitch *boundaries* will promote more opportunities (the designed-in affordances) related to the more technical intention, the development through exploration of the specific individual actions associated with generating *live* turnovers when pressing aggressively. In the second training camp, we made the decision to increase the number of *players* allocated to each team in the practices (6v6–7v7) to promote the players to *exploit* opportunities to press aggressively and create the need to work collectively when sealing the ball into the chosen area of the pitch. We also made the decision to provide the defensive team with an overload at certain points across the training camp. We feel like this additional player will provide defensive cover and promote the defensive team to be more aggressive and ultimately press more frequently. Although the trade-off coupled with providing this safety net needs to be considered, as the additional player may enable the defending team to seal the ball successfully into an area of the pitch using suboptimal actions that will be ineffective in the performance environment. It will be a judgement call by the coaching team of when to remove the additional defender if we feel we are getting the wrong side of the trade-off. In the final training camp, we decided to move the *player* numbers on each team to those more typical of the performance environment (8v8–11v11). The intention of the final training camp will be to develop the players' ability to employ and adapt appropriate systems of play and linked strategies to manufacture opportunities to press aggressively, the coaching team felt that this task required collective organisation of full (or close to full) playing teams. As a result of this the number of opportunities for each player to win the ball back is likely to be reduced, whilst this could be viewed as a limitation, we believe it will generate the need for the players to *execute* when the environment presents them with the opportunity.

The next *task* constraint for consideration is the *Ball Feed (location and frequency)*. We made the decision across all three training camps to slow the ball feed down by generating a pause prior to any dead ball restart in Zone 1 or Zone 2. With this task constraint manipulation we aim to initiate the cycle of co-adaptation between the defence and the attack across various phases. By slowing down the attacking phases we provide the opportunity for the defensive team to establish an organised defensive structure and remove any direct route to goal for the attacking team. This in turn will provoke the attacking team to enter into the process of destabilising the defensive system through a period of possession. This period of possession will offer the defending team the opportunity to step out of their defensive structure and press aggressively and thus becomes the designed-in affordance we want the players to interact with. It is important to note that the decision to slow the ball feed down does come with some negative trade-offs. The game of international hockey is played at a very high tempo. Therefore, the process of slowing the game down makes it less representative and has the potential to generate behaviours that will not be effective when playing the top teams. However, this is a limitation we are willing to tolerate in order to facilitate a greater frequency of the specific phase of the game linked to the session intention. We will ensure that within other practices throughout the training camps we will accelerate the ball feed to counteract this trade-off.

The final *task* constraint we have designed-in is the point scoring, *Point Scoring System (individual and team)*. Our initial thought process led us towards a point scoring system that rewarded the defensive team when they earnt a *live* turnover in Zone 3 or Zone 4. However, by considering the co-adaptive process, we anticipate that the attacking team will negate any opportunity for the defensive team to generate turnovers by playing the ball directly into Z1 and Z2. Whilst this would present an interesting problem for the defensive team to try and solve, it would work directly against us achieving the intention. We reflected and decided to take a subtler approach and kick-start the co-adaptation a phase earlier. By offering the attacking team a point reward for when one of their midfielders receives the ball in Z3, we anticipate that this will invite the defending team to step out aggressively and press to win the ball back rather than let the attacking team rack up a points total.

Coach Reflection – *As a coaching team we have learnt to initiate and subsequently steer the cycle of co-adaptation to meet our intentions. To kick-start this process of co-adaptation in training we start by manipulating the 'opposition' (in practice) or fellow team members (not directly linked to the session intention).*

In summary, we have explored the idea that practitioners at International-level sport need to consider how they *design-in* opportunities to interact with specifying information (task, opposition, pitch size) in order to support athletes to explore and nurture physical literacy. Using data to support this coaching intervention, we have explored how to reverse engineer specific landscapes rich in affordances and ensure that physical literacy is attended to within programme design. Whilst this remains a complex goal, the ability to promote functional movement skills through a wayfinding approach (as outlined in Chapter 2) might support our athletes as they develop intentional and motivated approaches to their performance development.

References

Araújo, D. & Davids, K. (2011). What exactly is acquired during skill acquisition?. *Journal of Consciousness Studies*, 18(3–4), 7–23.

Bloom, B. S. & Sosniak, L. A. (1985). *Developing talent in young people*. New York, NY: Ballantine Books.

Button, C., Seifert, L., Chow, J. Y., Davids, K. & Araujo, D. (2020). Dynamics of skill acquisition: An ecological dynamics approach. Champaign, IL: Human Kinetics Publishers.

Cannane, S. (2009). *First tests: Great Australian cricketers and the backyards that made them*. Sydney: ABC Books.

Connor, J. D., Farrow, D. & Renshaw, I. (2018). Emergence of skilled behaviors in professional, amateur and junior cricket batsmen during a representative training scenario. *Frontiers in Psychology*, 9(2012), https://doi.org/10.3389/fpsyg.2018.02012

Headrick, J., Renshaw, I., Davids, K., Pinder, R. A. & Araújo, D. (2015). The dynamics of expertise acquisition in sport: The role of affective learning design. *Psychology of Sport and Exercise*, 16, 83–90.

Hoggard., M. (2010). *Hoggy: Welcome to my world*. London: Harper-Collins.

Meyers, L. & Rowe, S. (2020). Complete Goalscoring Analysis & Comparison - Women's & Men's EuroHockey Championships 2019. https://www.myersandrowe.selz.com/

Phillips, E., Davids, K., Renshaw, I. & Portus, M. (2014). Acquisition of expertise in cricket fast bowling: Perceptions of expert players and coaches. *Journal of Science and Medicine in Sport*, 17(1), 85–90.

Renshaw, I. & Chappell, G. S. (2010). *A constraints-led approach to talent development in cricket*. In L. Kidman & B. Lombardo (Eds.), Athlete-centred coaching: Developing decision makers (2nd ed., pp. 151–173). Worcester, MA: IPC Print Resources.

Renshaw, I., Chappell, G. S., Fitzgerald, D. & Davison, J. (2010, 1–3 June 2010). The Battle Zone: Constraint-led coaching in action. Paper presented at the Conference of Science, Medicine & Coaching in Cricket, Sheraton Mirage, Gold Coast, Queensland, Australia.

Renshaw, I., Davids, K. & Savelsbergh, G. J. (Eds.). (2010). *Motor learning in practice: A constraints-led approach*. London: Routledge.

Renshaw, I., Davids, K., Newcombe, D. & Roberts, W. (2019). *The constraints led approach: Principles for sports coaching and practice design*. London: Routledge.

Roberts, W. M., Newcombe, D. J. & Davids, K. (2019). Application of a constraints-led approach to pedagogy in schools: Embarking on a journey to nurture physical literacy in primary physical education. *Physical Education and Sport Pedagogy*, 24(2), 162–175.

Weissensteiner, J., Abernethy, B., Farrow, D. & Müller, S. (2008). The development of anticipation: A cross-sectional examination of the practice experiences contributing to skill in cricket batting. *Journal of Sport and Exercise Psychology*, *30*(6), 663–684.

Whitehead, M. (2013). Definition of physical literacy and clarification of related issues. *ICSSPE Bulletin*, *65*(1.2).

13

MEASURING PHYSICAL LITERACY

A Fresh Approach

*Brett Wilkie, Jonathan Foulkes, James Rudd, Colin Lewis,
Carl Woods, Alice Sweeting and Ella Robinson*

13.1 Background

The main aim of this case study is to provide a novel tool to capture and measure physical literacy from an Ecological Dynamics conceptualisation. A secondary aim is to highlight that the current reductionist approach to the measurement of physical literacy is not appropriate to capture the embodied dimension of physical literacy.

13.2 The Dilemma of Continually Shifting Definitions of Physical Literacy

As outlined in Chapter 2, the original, and arguably most prominent, conceptualisation of physical literacy was put forward by Whitehead (2001), with a strong grounding in phenomenology. It is captured in Whitehead's (2001, p. 131) assertion that:

> A physically literate individual moves with poise, economy and confidence in a wide variety of physically challenging situations. The individual is perceptive in 'reading' all aspects of the physical environment, anticipating movement needs or possibilities and responding appropriately to these, with intelligence and imagination. Physical literacy requires a holistic engagement that encompasses physical capacities embedded in perception, experience, memory, anticipation and decision-making.

Since this conceptualisation, six further definitions have been put forward, with Whitehead's most recent definition describing physical literacy as *the motivation, confidence, physical competence, knowledge and understanding to value and take responsibility for engagement in physical activities for life* (IPLA, 2017). However, over the last 20 years, definitions of physical literacy have tended to move away from the importance of individual-environment interactions and how they shape physical literacy journeys, towards a reductionist and separate conceptualisation of the four overlapping and equally weighted constructs (as described above) that we need to teach children (Edwards et al., 2018). This shift has inevitably changed how practitioners and researchers engage with the concept of physical literacy.

13.3 Operationalised through Measurement

Across the globe, the common approach to measurement of physical literacy has been paradigmatically reductionist, tending to break down movements into discrete and quantifiable outcomes. For example, we continue to witness measurement of physical literacy focused on the quantification of separate physical, affective, and cognitive domains (Canadian approach); approximated scores, calculated from disconnected elements of physical, psychological, social, and cognitive skills (Australian approach); and checklists of set capabilities and achievements that every child should achieve (UK and Swedish approach). These approaches have a number of significant limitations for those who are looking at this concept from the point of view of Ecological Dynamics. Essentially, an Ecological Dynamics perspective would suggest that any attempt to deconstruct physical literacy into component parts and thus remove it from play, physical activity, or the performance environment is unlikely to provide an understanding of a child's physical literacy. This is because these systems interact and self-organise through movement and the context of play and physical activity is very different from the constraints acting on an individual in standardised assessment-based conditions.

13.4 Physical Literacy as a Process of Wayfinding

To capture physical literacy from an ecological dynamic approach it needs to be captured during play or in performance environments. Let us explore this through team invasion games which take place in highly dynamical environments (Davids, Button & Bennett, 2008). Informational constraints, such as the number and movement of defenders, the distance between teammates, changing score lines, and the duration of the game all enmesh to create unique and evolving problems as the game unfolds. Accordingly, setting out pre-determined 'plans' or tactical 'models of behaviour' rarely work, and trying to reduce the causes of behaviour down to one 'mechanism' discounts the non-linearity and dynamicity of a game (Ribeiro et al., 2019). Thus, any invasion game that a child is playing consists of dynamic problems that they must learn to solve by learning to perceive *ways* to exploit emerging gaps and spaces matched to their current action capabilities. This means that to understand a child's physical literacy when embedded in a games-based approach, we need to observe a child's movement skill in context, within the game. This can enable us to understand what information sources children attune to (i.e., detect), the affordances this information specifies to them and how they utilise these affordances to achieve task outcome(s). Subsequently, such an approach to viewing physical literacy requires an ecological epistemology, appreciating the mutual relationship between a child and their environment.

13.5 Understanding Learner-Environment Interactions during Games

When viewed through this lens, practitioners have the opportunity to collect new information and develop insight beyond what might otherwise be available through more traditional performance analysis tools. In this section, we explain how we generated a notational analysis through iteration, whereby potential performance indicators were introduced, discussed, trialled, and endorsed by technical experts within the field. The goal of the selected variables (shown in Tables 13.1–13.3) was to collect information on a

TABLE 13.1 On ball functionality and technical interactions – measurements and definitions

Interaction or behaviour	Description
Passing and shooting success	Categorises whether passes and shots were successful or unsuccessful. Where a successful pass is executed there is further evaluation to identify whether the pass was into contested or uncontested space.
Passing Direction	Categorises passes as penetrating, forward, lateral, defensive, or backwards.
Pass Length	Categorises passes as short, medium, or long.
Interaction Network	Identifies which player distributes the ball, and to whom the intended recipient is.

TABLE 13.2 Off ball offensive spatial-temporal interactions – measurements and definitions

Interaction or behaviour	Description
Movement into unoccupied space	Intentional movement to adopt a position currently unoccupied by opposition player(s) or teammate(s).
Movement into occupied space	Intentional movement to adopt a position that is occupied by a teammate(s).
Movement into contested space	Intentional movement to adopt a position that is occupied by opposition player(s).
Multiple offensive movements	Multiple intentional movements in response to changing game environment (e.g. having moved into unoccupied space that then becomes occupied resulting in the player adjusting their court/field position in recognition of being marked).
Movement results in becoming the target of a pass	Observed player becomes the intended target of a pass.
Network Interactions	Identifies whether observed player offers visual or verbal cues indicating their desire to be the target of the pass, is aware of the ball as evidenced by their scanning behaviours or is ignorant of the ball as evidenced by an absence of scanning behaviours directed to the ball.

TABLE 13.3 Off ball defensive spatial-temporal interactions – measurements and definitions

Interaction or behaviour	Description
Closing down player in possession	Intentional movement towards opponent in possession of the ball resulting in being the first player to apply pressure to the opposition player in possession. Court or pitch position also recorded.
Overloading player in possession	Intentional movement towards opponent in possession of the ball resulting in two defensive players applying pressure to the player in possession. Court or pitch position also recorded.
Swarming player in possession	Intentional movement towards opponent in possession of the ball resulting in three or more defensive players applying pressure to the player in possession. Court or pitch position also recorded.
(Defensive) Movement into unoccupied space	Intentional movement to adopt a position currently unoccupied by opposition player(s) or teammate(s).
(Defensive) Movement into contested space	Intentional movement to adopt a position that is occupied by opposition player(s)
Multiple defensive movements	Multiple intentional movements in response to changing game environment (e.g. having moved to mark a player initially the defensive player moves again as the attacking player adjusts their position).
Blocks or interception	Intentional movement that results in the defensive player attempting to, or successfully influencing the ball's movement through a tip, block, or interception.

range of learner-environment interactions (i.e., functionality of behaviour, and offensive and defensive temporo-spatial interactions). Observations framed in this manner allow insights into the learner's ability to attune to information and the affordances presented. For example, successfully identifying passing and shooting opportunities, effectively finding space, closing down opposition players, and implementing strategic patterns of play would allow us to build up a picture of an individual's knowledge of the environment and the affordances that the child is perceiving.

13.6 Bringing Life to This Analysis

Having introduced this notional analysis approach (presented in Tables 13.1–13.3), we will now show how it can be brought to life, using primary school-aged children participating in a commonly played, small-sided, conditioned, physical education game (mat ball). In the game, children were placed into teams of mixed movement ability based on their functional movement skill performance captured through the Dragons Challenge movement assessment (Stratton et al., 2015).[1] The court dimensions were 18m × 12m with a goal (a gym mat with a goalkeeper kneeling upon it) placed centrally at either end of the court. Games consisted of two, competitive, five-minute periods of play with a short break in the middle. Rules included: no-contact, no running with or dribbling of the ball, and scoring was only possible by shooting from within the opposition half.

This approach provided a more holistic evaluation and richer interpretation of physical literacy 'in action' than it is otherwise possible to obtain through reductionist assessments. Figures 13.1–13.3 display some indicative sample data representing an individual player's functionality and technical interactions data. These figures represent frequencies of pass direction, pass length, and the networks formed during the mat ball game. Table 13.4 provides a summary of the key differences that emerged from the notational analysis of gameplay behaviours and interactions.

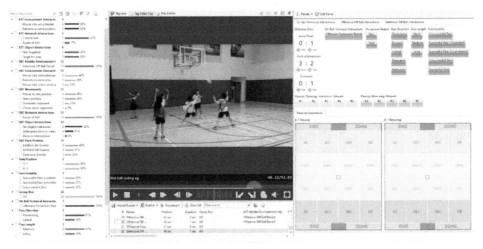

FIGURE 13.1 Dartfish tagging panel used to capture gameplay behaviours and learner-environment interactions

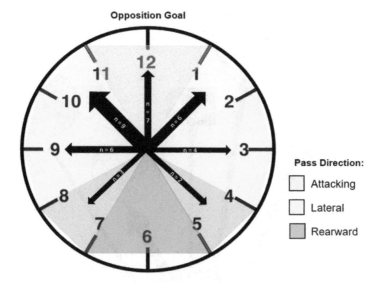

FIGURE 13.2 Analysis of Passing Direction data. The direction of the arrows indicates pass direction, and the width of the arrows denotes the frequency of passes in a particular direction (i.e., thicker arrows illustrate more passes)

13.7 How Physical Literacy Revealed Itself during Gameplay

A rich range of distinctive, thought-provoking, gameplay behaviours emerged from the analysis, highlighting what information in the environment children are self-regulating their action to. The tool proved sensitive enough to discern these subtler manifestations of this attunement and offered insights into the affordances that children were perceiving in the game. To supplement the summary data presented in Table 13.4, a range of indicative examples of observed games play are given to help illustrate the stark differences observed. Data showed that children with higher physical literacy and therefore *deeper knowledge of the environment* typically attempted more uncontested, attacking (penetrating or forward in direction) passes, over varied distances, compared to other players, regardless of the target player's physical literacy profile. Passing network data revealed children with higher levels of physical literacy also adopted *greater diversity in passing* and target identification than less physically literate individuals. Interestingly, the more physically literate players also demonstrated *greater capacity to regulate* their own court position based upon the player in possession of the ball, We saw the adoption of more advanced court positions, further from the ball when the player in possession was of higher physical literacy compared to reducing distance to the ball and demonstrating more overt visual and verbal signals of their availability as a target when possession was with less physically literate players. Defensive spatial-temporal behaviours indicated that swarming of the player in possession was a frequent off ball interaction for all learners irrespective of their knowledge of the environment. More physically literate players, whilst still demonstrating overload and swarming behaviours, however, did so with greater discretion. This demonstrated their ability to better regulate their behaviour so that swarming behaviours were more likely to be observed when they were in their own half, or in particular, when close to their own goal. Finally, those learners with greater physical literacy demonstrated a greater willingness to adjust

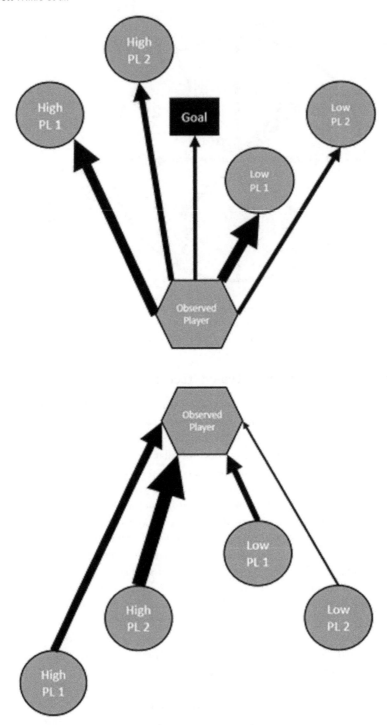

FIGURE 13.3 Analysis of Passing Networks data. The arrowhead and origin indicate individual children, with length and width of arrows indicating mean passing distance and frequency

TABLE 13.4 Frequency of observed gameplay behaviours. Very high ≥ 80% of observed behaviours, High = 60–79% of observed behaviours, Moderate = 40–59% of observed behaviours, Low = 20–39% of observed behaviours, Very low ≤ 20% of observed behaviours

Interaction or behaviour		Low physical literacy learners	High physical literacy learners	Difference comparing high to low literacy players
Passing success		Very high	Very high	No difference
Shooting success		Low	Moderate	Increased success
Direction of pass	Attacking	Very low	Moderate	More frequent
	Lateral	Moderate	Moderate	No difference
	Backwards	Moderate	Very low	Less frequent
Length of pass	Short	very high	Variable	Greater range of passing demonstrated
	Medium	very low		
	Long	very low		
Passing network		Seeks high physical literacy target	Balanced	Seeks variable targets
Offensive movement	Unoccupied space	Very low	Moderate	Moves into unoccupied space more frequently
	Occupied space	Low	Very low	Avoids moving into space occupied by team mates
	Contested space	Moderate	Low	Avoids moving into space occupied by opposition players
	Multiple movements	Very low	Low	More frequently demonstrates multiple movements
Network interactions	Visual cue offered	Moderate	High	More frequently indicates availability to receive pass
	Verbal cue offered	Very low	Moderate	More frequently shouts to receive pass
	Ball awareness	High	Very high	More frequently demonstrates ball tracking
Defensive movement	Closing down	Very low	Moderate	More frequently first defender to closing down
	Overloading	Moderate	Low	Less frequent overloading
	Swarming	Moderate	Very low	Less frequent swarming
	Unoccupied space	Very low	Very low	No difference
	Contested space	High	Moderate	Less frequently entered contested space
	Multiple movements	Very low	Moderate	More frequently adjusted position
	Blocks/interception	Very low	Very low	No difference

court position or defensive role associated with defensive off ball spatial-temporal inter-actions. If the physically literate learner was the second or third player to close down the player in possession, they were frequently recorded moving to an alternative court position as they sought to disrupt play with their newly adjusted defensive positioning. These secondary movements led to more frequent blocks and interceptions being attempted.

13.8 Conclusion

Undertaking an assessment that measures gameplay interactions enables researchers and practitioners to gain further insight into how learners effectively attune to the affordances offered within games and team activities. This case study provides a glimpse of a richer interpretation of physical literacy 'in action', that progresses understanding beyond what is offered through the isolated, reductionist examination of movement competence, confidence and knowledge and understanding. This is the first tool that we are aware of that taps into children's knowledge of the environment. We hope that the opportunity to acquire such uniquely original insight will stimulate practitioners and researchers to renounce mass measurement and embrace a move towards the assessment of physical literacy through embodied learner-environment interactions in naturalistic settings.

Note

1 Children completed a small movement circuit, called the 'Dragon Challenge' that allowed us to assess their movement competence. The circuit takes children approximately 90–240 seconds to complete and consists of locomotor, balance and object control tasks such as sprinting, walking over a balance beam and dribbling a basketball. Each circuit was video recorded in order to allow each child's performance to be assessed by a trained assessor at a later date. A Dragon Challenge score (0–54) i.e. continuous data, is created for each child by totalling the scores from three assessment criteria, these being technique (0–18) looking at how competently children carried out each skill; outcome (0–18) focusing on whether the skill outcome was met or not and finally; time (0–18) namely, the time it took the child to complete the course. (https://www.youtube.com/watch?v=lSPLtwDrgRM)

References

Davids, K. W., Button, C. & Bennett, S. J. (2008). *Dynamics of skill acquisition: A constraints-led approach.* Champaign, IL: Human Kinetics.

Edwards, L. C., Bryant, A. S., Keegan, R. J., Morgan, K., Cooper, S. M. & Jones, A. M. (2018). 'Measuring' physical literacy and related constructs: A systematic review of empirical findings *Sports Medicine, 48*(3), 659–682.

International Physical Literacy Association. (2017). International Physical Literacy Association. Retrieved from https://www.physical-literacy.org.uk/

Ribeiro, J. F., Davids, K., Araújo, D., Guilherme, J., Silva, P., Garganta, J. (2019). Exploiting bi-directional self-organising tendencies in team sports: The role of the game model and tactical principles of play. *Frontiers in Psychology, 10,* 2213.

Stratton, G., Foweather, L., Rotchell, J., English, J., Hughes, H. (2015). *Dragon challenge V1. 0 Manual.* Cardiff: Sport Wales.

Whitehead, M. (2001). The concept of physical literacy. *European Journal of Physical Education, 6,* 127–138.

14

DEVELOPMENT OF CREATIVE MOVEMENT THROUGH ENRICHED GAME DESIGN

Ella Robinson, Colin Lewis, James Rudd, Jonathan Foulkes, Brett Wilkie, Carl Woods and Alice Sweeting

14.1 Movement Creativity

Creative, adaptive movements are generally defined as a functional and original action solution to achieve an intended task goal (Hristovski et al., 2011; Orth et al., 2017). As emphasised throughout this book, within an Ecological Dynamics approach, movement emerges from a continuous, cyclical and prospective coupling of perception, cognition and action, situated in the dynamic performer-environment interaction(s) (Gibson, 1979; Davids, Handford & Williams, 1994; Warren, 2006). Humans move to perceive what opportunities for action their environment offers, perceiving surrounding affordances to (self) organise their actions (Michaels & Beek, 1995; Bruineberg & Rietveld, 2014). Across the surrounding affordance landscape, some affordances stand out and invite performers to certain actions (Bruineberg & Rietveld, 2014). For example, within a school gym, placing a line of cones on the ground invites intentionality for most children to weave, forwards, in and out of the cones. However, creative interactions with the cones can emerge over time through a transformational process, inviting search, exploration and discovery of novel and functionally efficient actions (Hristovski, Davids & Araujo, 2009; for example in dance improvisation, see Kimmel, Hristova & Kussmaul, 2018; Rudd et al., 2020). Through exploratory behaviours, humans have opportunities and capacities to adapt creative movements to achieve the same or different goals (Hristovski, Davids & Araujo, 2009). Due to the human body's ability to flexibly switch between different movement patterns due to it being a multi-stable, degenerate system (Kelso, 2012; Seifert, Button & Davids, 2013), the more enriched an environment and greater the action capabilities of an individual, the higher the possibilities for movement innovations and adaptations through interaction with objects, surfaces, ledges, inclines and other individuals. As a result, this will help to create abundance of movement options.

14.2 Movement Creativity: A Tricky Affair

Prompting the emergence of creativity can be a tricky affair, as people, typically, are attracted to and utilise affordances to guide their movement that are socially or historically accepted in their societies (O'Sullivan et al., 2020). In other words, they model their

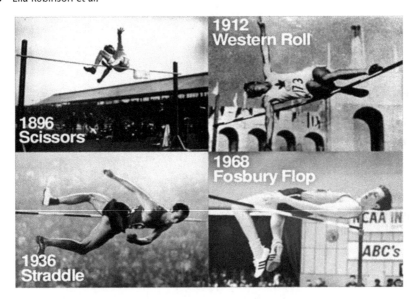

FIGURE 14.1 The evolution of high jump technique from 1896 to 1968 (Mayooshin, 2017)

actions, following norms and seeking to imitate actions of icons, do what is typically done and act within their comfort zone. For example, if a teacher turns on the music during a physical education (PE) class and asks the children to dance, anecdotally, they will all likely perform a handful of dance movements, which correspond to the current "hits," e.g., "the floss dance" (see https://www.youtube.com/watch?v=gaEbJ4ShH3U). Designing learning environments for creativity to emerge requires the exposure of learners to a broad range of task constraints and affordances, as well as a safe space to encourage an individual to continuously explore functional and novel movement solutions. For example, in teaching the high jump, the introduction of foam-safety mats revolutionised the high jump technique, due to the mats acting as a constraint for the safe exploration and practice of landing on the back, promoting the emergence of a new, creative and highly functional movement solution – the "Fosbury Flop (see Figure 14.1)."

In high-performance sport and PE settings, coaches and teachers are considered environmental designers who can influence learners' intentions and invite them to explore and discover possibilities for a range of creative movements to emerge from their interactions with the lesson surrounds and layout. What might these enriched environments for inducing opportunities for innovative and adaptive movements look like within PE settings? In this case study, we will explore how practitioners can manipulate constraints to promote exploration, allowing for creativity to emerge, outlining a method for measuring movement creativity and setting out an experimental design across the respective settings.

14.3 Exploring Enriched Environments

A key message of this book is that sustainable engagement in physical activity and enhancement of physical literacy can be induced by "enrichment" activities for learners: the design of a rich variation of athletic, participatory experiences, opportunities, challenges and activities that will require skill adaptation (Button et al., 2020). Indeed, the external agent (e.g., coach, teacher) is the designer who can manipulate lesson constraints with the intent of improving the learner's capabilities to explore and discover creative actions. In a range of different movement contexts, practitioners can manipulate constraints to promote exploration by making changes to the environment through careful planning and design of the environment. However, we acknowledge that affordances are always available in an environment. Therefore, although practitioners should not expect children to come up with the same movement solutions, the value and meanings of affordances change, depending on the skills and capacities the child already possesses (effectivities) (Davids, Araujo & Brymer, 2016). As we note below, high-performance sport and PE settings are ideal locations for enrichment to evolve.

14.4 Supporting Physical Literacy in Our Children: Designing Creativity in High-Performance Sport

Considering the context of football (soccer), an example of enrichment could be implemented in a simple playing out from the back activity, requiring players to play out the ball from their defensive end of the pitch, whereby the goalkeeper starts with the ball and players are then tasked with retaining possession as they progress the ball through the key areas of the pitch. In this activity, a coach could provide a highly rigid structure by assigning players specific positions, or zones, to inhabit on the pitch, and further prescribing roles for individual players. What is problematic with rigid designs such as this, is that they will not, and do not, afford creativity to emerge. This is due to the design of the learning environment providing little information for players to interact with, which can result in fewer opportunities to explore different innovative and adaptive movement solutions, and a typical over-emphasis on repetition of the coach, or teacher, prescribed movement solutions (Vaughan, Mallet & Davids, 2019). This information is often captured in sequential teaching points for instructors e.g., steps 1–4 in receiving a pass, looking up, making a decision and passing the ball. Instead, to support exploration and discovery of creative solutions that might emerge, the coach could enhance the information available, by manipulating the constraints of the environment (e.g., adding opposition players, changing the dimensions of the playing area, adding conditions to the game) or the equipment (e.g., adding another ball or goal to aim for). As a result, the learning environment will now offer a greater number and range of affordances, inviting players to explore and discover novel actions, in the search for efficient movement solutions (Hristovski, Davids & Araujo, 2009). Fewer prescriptive verbal instructions will be provided and may be limited to guiding the search of the learner not prescribing solutions. This type of learning design will facilitate many opportunities for learners to experience the coupling of perception, cognition and action, during their interactions with the environment and the game constraints.

14.5 Supporting Physical Literacy in Our Children: Designing Creativity into Youth Sport Activities

14.5.1 The Game of Gateways

In youth sport, a game that can be used by teachers and coaches is the game of Gateways. Gateways is a game during which participants are required to travel through as many gates as they can in 4 minutes. Normally, a gate is set up by placing two cones 1 m apart to form a gateway for the children to move through. Once set up is complete, the children will play the game, being active and hopefully having fun. Based on the work conducted by Araújo et al. (2004) and Davids, Button & Bennett (2008) on Ecological Dynamics, we understand that adaptive behaviour, rather than being imposed by a pre-existing structure, emerges from this confluence of constraints under the boundary condition of a particular task or goal (Araújo et al., 2009). Therefore, individuals take advantage of the informational richness of environmental properties, thus, learning occurs when there are changes in the environmental properties to which perceptual systems are sensitive (Jacobs & Michaels, 2007).

14.5.2 Designing Gateways Based upon an Ecological Dynamics Conceptualisation of Physical Literacy

First, let us reflect on the environment created in a standard game of Gateways. As demonstrated in Figure 14.2, cones are placed in a symmetrical structure to form rows and columns of gates. If we consider the thoughts of Jacobs and Michaels (2007), informational richness within a symmetrical environment is limited, providing fewer opportunities for children to cleverly perceive and utilise many affordances of the environment. Another consideration for the teacher is their instructions and how these will constrain creativity, an example of a commonly used instruction would be:

> Today we are going to play a game called Gateways. You will have X minutes to run through as many gates as you can. Ready, off we go!

Notice here how the instructions for the task by the practitioner directly tells the children to "run" instead of "move." Therefore, the movement patterns produced are likely to be repetitive solutions, lacking in creativity. A clever practitioner needs to think enrichment

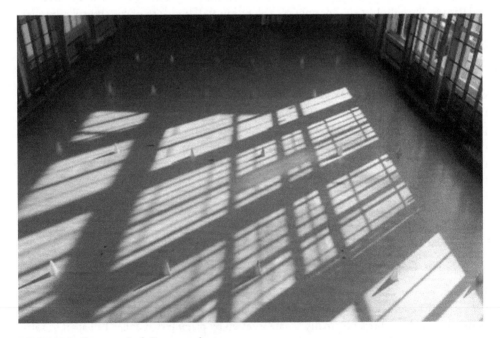

FIGURE 14.2 Symmetrical Gateways layout

of the game Gateways is necessary to afford greater opportunities for learning through the emergence of creative movement.

14.5.3 Re-designing Gateways to Develop Movement Creativity

Can Gateways be re-designed as a game to develop movement creativity during children's play? Following on from the symmetrical structure, implementation of an asymmetrical design catered for greater exploration of the environment. This design, pictured in Figure 14.3, is constructed by re-positioning the gates still 1 m apart, the gates are also of different colours and placed at various angles throughout the vicinity of the playing area. However, whilst this further exploration is welcomed, there will not necessarily be new self-organisation of movement patterns. This is because there is limited new information, rather just a change in the positioning of the gates and colours. Therefore, participants may still be restricted in opportunities for action.

In order to develop the opportunities for greater affordances, the instructions given by the coach or teacher could be adapted to encourage self-regulation of functional movement solutions. For instance, amending the word "run" to "move" should invite children to explore and discover novel and functionally efficient actions:

> Today we are going to play a game called Gateways. The aim of the game is to find as many different gates as you can, and move through them in as many different ways as you can. You will have X minutes to play the game. Ready, off we go.

Building on this re-design feature, we can enrich the environment further by adapting gates using equipment (e.g., climbing frames, gymnastics vaults, benches, balance beams). Adding this equipment creates a super-rich environment, pictured in Figure 14.4, with

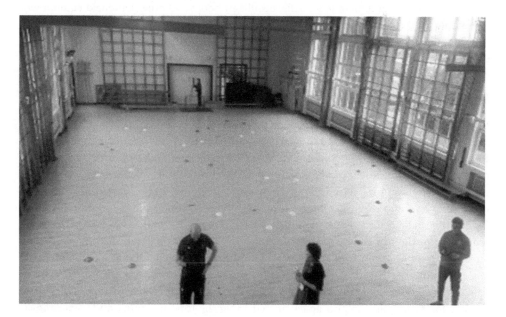

FIGURE 14.3 Asymmetrical Gateways layout

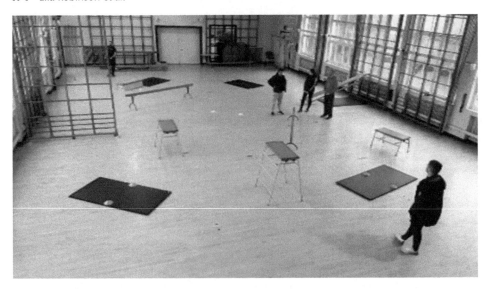

FIGURE 14.4 Super-rich Gateways layout

extra information that affords further opportunities for the development of creative movement. Specifically, this is because the child is able to perceive information from, and explore, a wider variety of equipment and different planes/axis of movement, whilst having the challenge of producing innovative movement solutions. It is also worth noting that this layout is starting to resemble a parkour installation. Indoor parkour environments have the potential to promote creative and exploratory movement behaviours, through heightened opportunities for decision-making and action functionality (Rudd et al., 2020). What is also of particular interest, is that this exploratory movement can be performed with or without a piece of equipment (e.g., balls, beanbags, hoops and other handheld equipment), depending on the constraints issued by the practitioner. Again, manipulating the nature of the equipment available to the children will ensure affordances stand out, soliciting children to perform various actions.

14.6 Assessment Using Gateways for Researchers and Practitioners

Using a form of assessment to measure creativity will enable researchers and practitioners to observe and better appreciate the need for enrichment of high-performance sport and PE settings. A form of assessment will be able to demonstrate to the external agent (coach, teacher, participant(s)), the development of skills/creative movements over a period of time, across the various environments. To measure creativity, we would recommend using our example of measuring flexibility, innovation and persistence (defined in Table 14.1). Flexibility can be recorded by scoring a point each time a new skill is observed in a child's repertoire for the first time when moving through a gate. Innovation can be recorded by scoring a point each time a skill is performed innovatively when moving through a gate (e.g., in a different direction or using a different body part). Persistence can be calculated using the flexibility score divided by the innovation score for each skill. The overall persistence for each child can also be calculated using the total flexibility and total innovative solutions. As an example, when observing development, if the child's flexibility and

TABLE 14.1 Measurement definitions for scoring creativity (adapted from Lenetsky et al., 2015 and Moraru, Memmert & van der Kamp, 2016)

Measurement	Definition
Innovation	Total number of different solutions that emerge when performing the same functional movement skill, such as using different body parts to perform similar thematic movements (e.g., jumping 1–2 feet, 2–2 feet, 2–1 foot, using 1 arm, 2 feet).
Flexibility	The total number of different functional movement solutions observed.
Persistence	The average number of movement solutions that originate from the same category. Determined by dividing the Flexibility score by the Innovation (also known as Fluency) score.

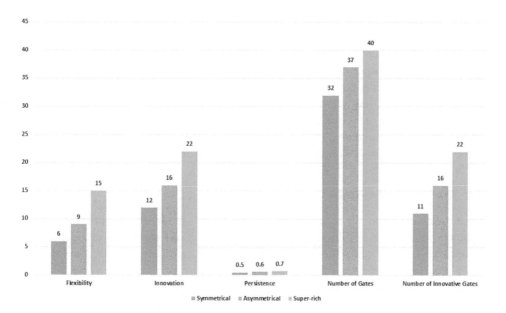

FIGURE 14.5   Example data from scoring system for measuring creativity

innovation scores are higher in the super-rich environment, in comparison to that of the symmetrical, then the practitioner can assume the child has used a wider variety of creative movement solutions. In addition, the number of gates and innovative gates that a child moves through can also be recorded. See Figure 14.5 for an example of a child's creative measurements across a symmetrical, asymmetrical and super-rich environment.

To help with the scoring, video recordings can be used as an analytical tool by practitioners to retrospectively score each child using the proposed scoring system, to assist our understanding of movement and creativity (Rudd et al., 2020).

14.7 Experimental Design for the Game of Gateways

We would now like to signpost practitioners to an experimental design that can be implemented in their own contexts. We consider the creation of an experimental design valuable and in the best interests of a coach or teacher, given the prospect of being able to explore how creativity emerges under different environmental conditions. In turn, this

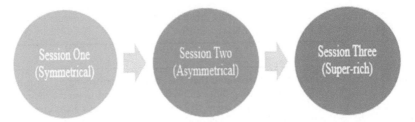

FIGURE 14.6 Experimental design for the delivery of Gateways

approach could then impact future coaching/teaching practice and inform how practitioners can manipulate constraints to promote exploration, allowing for creativity to emerge. The recommended experimental design would involve a three-session activity plan (see Figure 14.6), which uses each of the three environments on a rotational basis. To ensure each environment is explored, session one would be symmetrical, session two asymmetrical and session three super-rich. Once more, this will allow the external agents to detect the development of skills/creative movements over a period of time. We would expect to see little creativity in the symmetrical environment, slightly increased creativity in the asymmetrical environment and a significant increase in the creative movements in the super-rich environment, due to enriched environments providing more information to the participants, affording more opportunities for movement solutions.

14.8 Take-Home Messages

Within this case study, we have defined and discussed affordances or opportunities for action that emerge during creative movements. As explained, this is challenging for coaches and teachers in high-performance sport and PE settings, given the societal pressures placed on children to copy, imitate, rehearse and repeat in order to perform the "norm," movement patterns commonly accepted in society. What we have suggested is, exploring enriched environments through manipulating constraints can be beneficial to highlighting an extensive number and range of available affordances, encouraging children to read the environment and develop functional movement solutions. We must note that affordances are always available in an environment. However, their value and meaning change depending on the individual's effectivities. We recommend a scoring system and experimental design, incorporating environmental (symmetrical, asymmetrical and super-rich) and equipment (cones, balls, beanbags, hoops) manipulation, to endeavour to the enrichment of game-design. We envisage that researchers and practitioners who act upon the take-home messages of this case study, will be able to inform their own scholarly activity or practice, to better understand and implement enriched environments for children, to enhance movement creativity, within high-performance sport and PE settings.

References

Araújo, D., Davids, K., Bennett, S., Button, C. & Chapman, G. (2004). Emergence of sport skills under constraints. In *Skill acquisition in sport: Research, theory and practice*. London: Routledge.

Araujo, D., Davids, K. W., Chow, J. Y. & Passos, P. (2009). The development of decision making skill in sport: An ecological dynamics perspective. In M. Raab, D. Araujo & H. Ripoll (Eds.), *Perspectives on cognition and action in sport* (pp. 157–169). United States: Nova Science Publishers, Inc.

Bruineberg, J. & Rietveld, E. (2014). Self-organization, free energy minimization, and optimal grip on a field of affordances. *Frontiers in Human Neuroscience*, *8*, 599. doi:10.3389/fnhum.2014.00599.

Button, C., Seifert, L., Chow, J. Y., Davids, K. & Araujo, D. (2020). Dynamics of skill acquisition: An ecological dynamics approach. Champaign, IL: Human Kinetics Publishers.

Davids, K., Araujo, D. & Brymer, E. (2016). Designing affordances for physical activity: An ecological dynamics perspective. *Sports Medicine*, *46*, 933–938. doi:10.1007/s40279-016-0511-3.

Davids, K. W., Button, C. & Bennett, S. J. (2008). Dynamics of skill acquisition: A constraints-led approach. Champaign, IL: Human Kinetics.

Davids, K., Handford, C. & Williams, M. (1994). The natural physical alternative to cognitive theories of motor behaviour: an invitation for interdisciplinary research in sports science? *Journal of Sports Sciences*, *12*, 495–528. doi:10.1080/02640419408732202.

Gibson, J. J. (1979). *The ecological approach to visual perception*. Boston, MA: Houghton, Mifflin and Company.

Hristovski, R., Davids, K. W. & Araujo, D. (2009). Information for regulating action in sport: Metastability and emergence of tactical solutions under ecological constraints. In *Perspectives on Cognition and Action in Sport* (pp. 43–57). New York: Nova Science Publishers Inc.

Hristovski, R., Davids, K., Araujo, D. & Passos, P. (2011). Constraints-induced emergence of functional novelty in complex neurobiological systems: a basis for creativity in sport. *Nonlinear Dynamics – Psychology and Life Sciences*, *15*(2), 175.

Jacobs, D. M. & Michaels, C. F. (2007). Direct learning. *Ecological Psychology*, *19*(4), 321–349.

Kelso, J. S. (2012). Multistability and metastability: understanding dynamic coordination in the brain. *Philosophical Transactions of the Royal Society B: Biological Sciences*, *367*(1591), 902–918.

Kimmel, M., Hristova, D. & Kussmaul, K. (2018). Sources of embodied creativity: Interactivity and ideation in contact improvisation. *Behavioral Sciences*, *8*(6), 52.

Lenetsky, S., Nates, R. J., Brughelli, M. & Harris, N. K. (2015). Is effective mass in combat sports punching above its weight? *Human Movement Science*, *40*, 89–97.

Mayooshin.com (2017). The Dick Fosbury flop: How to think outside the box and innovate new ideas [online]. Available at: https://www.mayooshin.com/dick-fosbury/ Accessed on: 3rd August 2020.

Michaels, C. & Beek, P. (1995). The state of ecological psychology. *Ecological Psychology*, *7*(4), 259–278.

Moraru, A., Memmert, D. & van der Kamp, J. (2016). Motor creativity: the roles of attention breadth and working memory in a divergent doing task. *Journal of Cognitive Psychology*, *28*(7), 856–867.

Orth, D., van der Kamp, J., Memmert, D. & Savelsbergh, G. J. P. (2017). Creative motor actions as emerging from movement variability. *Journal of Frontiers in Psychology*, *8*, 1–8. Retrieved from https://www.frontiersin.org/articles/10.3389/fpsyg.2017.01903/full

O'Sullivan M, Davids, K., Woods CT, Rothwell M. & Rudd J. (2020). Conceptualizing physical literacy within an ecological dynamics framework. *Quest*. doi:10.1080/00336297.2020.1799828.

Rudd, J. R., Pesce, C., Strafford, B. W. & Davids, K. (2020). Physical literacy-A journey of individual enrichment: An ecological dynamics rationale for enhancing performance and physical activity in all. *Frontiers in Psychology*, *11*, 1904. doi:10.3389/fpsyg.2020.01904.

Seifert, L., Button, C. & Davids, K. (2013). Key properties of expert movement systems in sport. *Sports Medicine*, *43*(3), 167–178.

Seifert, L., Wattebled, L., L'Hermette, M., Bideault, G., Herault, R. & Davids, K. (2013). Skill transfer, affordances and dexterity in different climbing environments. *Human Movement Science*, *32*(6), 1339–1352.

Sport Australia. (2019). Physical Literacy. Retrieved from https://www.sportaus.gov.au/physical_literacy

Sport England. (2016). New plan to get children active. Retrieved from https://www.sportengland.org/news/government-launch-school-sport-and-activity-action-plan

Vaughan, J., Mallet, C. J. & Davids, K. (2019). Developing creativity to enhance human potential in sport: a wicked transdisciplinary challenge. *Sheffield Hallam University Research Archive*, 2090. Retrieved from https://www.frontiersin.org/articles/10.3389/fpsyg.2019.02090/full?utm_source=F-NTF&utm_medium=EMLX&utm_campaign=PRD_FEOPS_20170000_ARTICLE

Warren, W. H. (2006). The dynamics of perception and action. *Psychological Review*, *113*, 358. doi:10.1037/0033-295X.113.2.358.

INDEX